Continuing Professional Development in Health and Social Care

Continuing Professional Development in Health and Social Care

Strategies for Lifelong Learning

SECOND EDITION

Auldeen Alsop, EdD

Emeritus Professor
Sheffield Hallam University
Sheffield, UK

WILEY-BLACKWELL

A John Wiley & Sons, Ltd., Publication

This edition first published 2013 © 2013 by John Wiley & Sons Ltd.

Wiley-Blackwell is an imprint of John Wiley & Sons, formed by the merger of Wiley's global Scientific, Technical and Medical business with Blackwell Publishing.

Registered office: John Wiley & Sons, Ltd, The Atrium, Southern Gate, Chichester, West Sussex, PO19 8SQ, UK

Editorial offices: 9600 Garsington Road, Oxford, OX4 2DQ, UK
The Atrium, Southern Gate, Chichester, West Sussex, PO19 8SQ, UK
111 River Street, Hoboken, NJ 07030-5774, USA

For details of our global editorial offices, for customer services and for information about how to apply for permission to reuse the copyright material in this book please see our website at www.wiley.com/wiley-blackwell.

Library of Congress Cataloging-in-Publication Data

Alsop, Auldeen.
   Continuing professional development in health and social care ; strategies for lifelong learning / Auldeen Alsop. – 2nd ed.
      p. ; cm.
   Rev. ed. of: Continuing professional development / Auldeen Alsop. 2000.
   Includes bibliographical references and index.
   ISBN 978-1-4443-3790-7 (pbk. : alk. paper) – ISBN 978-1-118-53954-5 (emobi) – ISBN 978-1-118-53955-2 (epdf) – ISBN 978-1-118-53956-9 (epub)
   I. Alsop, Auldeen. Continuing professional development.   II. Title.
   [DNLM: 1. Allied Health Personnel–education.   2. Education, Continuing.
3. Professional Competence. W 18]
   615.8′5150715–dc23

                                                                        2012043160

A catalogue record for this book is available from the British Library.

Wiley also publishes its books in a variety of electronic formats. Some content that appears in print may not be available in electronic books.

Cover image: Shutterstock image 15995926 © vanias
Cover design by Sandra Heath

Set in 10/12.5pt Times by Aptara® Inc., New Delhi, India
Printed and bound in Malaysia by Vivar Printing Sdn Bhd

1   2013

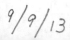

Contents

Preface   vi
Acknowledgements   ix

1   **Lifelong learning and continuing professional development**   1

2   **Regulation of allied health and social care professionals**   12

3   **The professional portfolio**   22

4   **The process of continuing professional development**   34

5   **Learning to learn**   47

6   **Learning with others**   58

7   **Learning in the workplace**   68

8   **Scholarly activity and research for the practitioner**   84

9   **Learning to write and writing to learn**   101

10   **Career development**   114

11   **CPD and career development for academics**   125

12   **Leadership and professional development**   136

13   **Learning strategies and CPD for support workers**   146

14   **Learning for leisure and pleasure**   153

Index   159

Preface

A considerable number of changes have occurred with regard to the regulation of health care professionals and the environment in which they work since the publication of the earlier book on continuing professional development (Alsop, 2000). The new regulatory body for allied health professionals in the United Kingdom, the Health Professions Council (HPC), was established on 1 April 2002, superseding the Council for Professions Supplementary to Medicine (CPSM) that had been in place since 1960. More stringent criteria for the regulation of the existing 12 professions came into force with the advent of the HPC. Over time, the HPC set up standards of education and training, standards of proficiency for each profession, standards of conduct, performance and ethics and standards for continuing professional development for the allied health professions. Over the last 10 years, a number of other professions have been admitted to the HPC register after fulfilling the strict criteria for entry. A more significant change came in August 2012 when social workers were admitted on to the register and the HPC (after legal ratification) changed its name to the Health and Care Professions Council (HCPC) to reflect the new mix of registered professions. The number of professions now regulated by the HCPC is 16, and no further entrants are expected. All changes since 2002 have placed significantly more responsibility on the regulated practitioners to take steps to maintain their competence to practise.

The regulation of health and social care practitioners in other countries has also seen some changes, particularly in Australia. South Africa has had its own HPC for some time. The United States and Canada have licensing systems that differ from state to state or province to province. Australia has recently moved to a national regulatory system for the professions involved in delivering health care. Across the world, the range of health care professions that fall within the remit of a body responsible for regulation varies from country to country. All now have similar requirements for the maintenance of competence. Some countries such as Australia and South Africa also include students in their scheme.

Just as changes have occurred in regulation, changes have also taken place in the employment context in which health and social care professionals practise, particularly in the United Kingdom. Developments in technology and other working practices and financial constraints on service provision have required the professions to do things differently and more autonomously. Being able to deal with change is certainly on the agenda. No longer is the National Health Service (NHS) the only significant employer of health care professionals. New working environments and new business arrangements are being established that enable professionals to develop practices that meet the needs of service users in very different ways and in a variety of markets. Some new businesses and social enterprises have been formed by entrepreneurial professionals. Some have contracts with the NHS and some offer services directly to the public. In the coming years, more of these services may well be established, offering more choices to service users and more directly meeting their needs.

These changes clearly impact on the ways in which health and social care practitioners now need to function. As Barnett (1994) has always advocated, professionals must be prepared to examine society's changing demands and take steps to shape change, embracing new practices and discarding outdated ones. It is important for professionals to have vision and be proactive in offering new types of services that meet current and future needs as changes continue to occur for the context of practice. Professional education has to prepare practitioners to develop new skills and qualities to meet changing demands. This is relevant not only for students of the professions but also for the professionals in practice. New schemes for continuing professional development need to be developed to reflect the changes in practice and to enable practitioners to develop the skills to operate in the new environments. Business skills in particular are required to support practitioners in developing very different career profiles and to use their talents and skills creatively in a different way. As career opportunities in public services wane for some health professionals, other opportunities become available. Professionals must thus make very different decisions about the ways in which their career might progress and prepare themselves by developing new skill sets for new opportunities in practice.

Although new requirements regarding professional regulation and maintenance of competence have provided the impetus for continuing professional development, a much wider perspective on learning should also be taken. Lifelong learning embraces improvement of knowledge, skill and personal competence in order to participate actively within society across the lifespan and not just in working life. Therefore, this text addresses the broader remit of lifelong learning, of which continuing professional development is an associated part. Given the fast-changing nature of employment in health and social care, professionals are advised not to limit their development activities to those meeting the requirements of the regulatory body. Instead, they should take a wider view of their personal development and maximise their skills and capacity to take advantage of new employment and career opportunities as they arise. Therefore, learning should take on a different meaning and not focus exclusively on the requirements of the regulatory body.

Learning is an adventure. Learning takes us from the known to the unknown in order to enhance our knowledge further. Reflection helps us make sense of otherwise senseless situations and helps us make links between otherwise disparate entities. Learning brings the previously impossible towards the potentially possible and generates a better sense of self and self-belief in the process. Learning can be risky. Learning can be fun. Learning can transform us. It depends on the way in which learning experiences are allowed to challenge or guide us. As Souza de Freitas (2007, p. xxvi) suggested in her Foreword to Paulo Freire's work *Daring to Dream: Toward a Pedagogy of the Unfinished*, 'to dream is to imagine horizons of possibilities'. She reinforced Freire's argument of the need to find joy in learning through curiosity and creative imagination. After all, imagination (according to Einstein) is more important than knowledge (Park, 2007).

Thus, the venture in this book is to focus once more on learning and learning opportunities in the widest possible sense. The current political climate now requires us as individuals to take more responsibility for our own development, our lifelong learning and our work and career efforts, in very uncertain times. The responsibility has been firmly passed to us to take steps to become fit for a place in the workforce, to maintain and develop that fitness and to contribute to society. Those with professional careers have even more obligations with regard to public safety and for demonstrating ongoing fitness to practise in the professional role. Steps have to be taken to sustain competence. This demands energy, initiative, inspiration, imagination and organisation. It requires constant attention to the potential of ad hoc learning opportunities and a creative approach to developing and using opportunities that can meet needs, targets and aspirations. This book addresses the issues of informal and formal learning and provides ideas for personal and professional development that not only keep professionals fit to practise but also stretch their imagination so as to fulfil personal dreams. The earlier edition of this book also referred to ways of making dreams a reality. Success in any venture means building self-esteem, setting demanding goals, always being positive, establishing good habits, mastering the art of communication, learning from role models, thriving under pressure, being persistent, learning from adversity and surviving success. Engaging in lifelong learning and not just in the essential development activity to maintain competence in the job brings more choices and more opportunities to diversify and maintain meaningful employment throughout the lifespan. Learning for leisure and pleasure ensures a meaningful life beyond the work role and into retirement.

References

Alsop A (2000) *Continuing Professional Development: A Guide for Therapists*. Blackwell Science, Oxford.

Barnett R (1994) *The Limits of Competence: Knowledge, Higher Education and Society*. The Society for Research into Higher Education & Open University Press, Buckingham.

Park P (2007) Foreword. In: *Daring to Dream: Toward a Pedagogy of the Unfinished* (ed. P Freire), pp xxxi–xxxvii. Paradigm Publishers, Boulder, CO.

Souza de Freitas AL (2007) Foreword. In: *Daring to Dream: Toward a Pedagogy of the Unfinished* (ed. P Freire), pp xxx–xxxiii. Paradigm Publishers, Boulder, CO.

Acknowledgements

I would particularly like to thank Zoë Parker, Education Manager (Lifelong Learning) at the College of Occupational Therapists, London, for her ongoing support and advice during the preparation of this book. Zoë has spent significant amount of time reading and giving invaluable feedback on draft chapters. In the course of writing the book, Zoë and I have developed a friendship that is reflected in Chapter 6, in the piece on critical kinship, to which she made a particular contribution. I would also like to acknowledge the guidance I have received from Professor Martin Rice, University of Toledo, USA; Professor Susan Ryan, University of Newcastle, Australia; and my colleagues at the University of Alberta, Canada, and at the University of Cape Town, South Africa. All have provided insights into their regulatory and continuing professional development systems. Finally, I should like to thank Claire Craig for her contributions through many critical discussions about practice and particularly with regard to the use of technology.

Auldeen Alsop

Chapter 1

Lifelong learning and continuing professional development

This chapter addresses:

1. lifelong learning as an underpinning philosophy for all personal learning and development;
2. the nature of employment and competent performance in practice;
3. definitions and meaning of continuing professional development.

Introduction

The Preface of this book sets out the premise on which this book is written. The Preface acknowledges the need for health and social care professionals to remain competent in the work that they do and thus to be able to undertake their work with service users competently and confidently within the constraints of an ever-challenging and ever-changing health and social care environment. However, this is only part of the story as the Preface advocates learning to fulfil wider ambitions throughout life. This chapter is first and foremost concerned with lifelong learning, a notion that is more wide-ranging than continuing professional development (CPD). This chapter sets the scene for CPD by first offering a more liberal view of lifelong learning as an underpinning philosophy for all personal learning and development. It establishes lifelong learning as a highly desirable activity for everyone regardless of any legal responsibilities that come with being a health or social care professional. This chapter explores the advantages of taking personal responsibility for engaging in development activities for life.

Later chapters in this book explore the rationale for CPD in both a legal and professional sense and address various ways in which competence to practise can be both maintained and advanced. It is worth looking beyond the constraints of the legal requirements in order to explore the nature of learning and the advantages it

Continuing Professional Development in Health and Social Care: Strategies for Lifelong Learning,
Second Edition. Auldeen Alsop.
© 2013 John Wiley & Sons, Ltd. Published 2013 by John Wiley & Sons, Ltd.

brings within a lifetime. Lifelong learning activities thus become personally desirable and meaningful activities rather than selected activities to confirm ongoing fitness to practise. This book offers a source of information for all those wishing to learn to improve their career prospects and develop their competence for new roles and responsibilities in their field of work or wider career. First, there is a need to explore lifelong learning as a background to all aspects of life in support of employment and career enhancement.

Lifelong learning

The concept of lifelong learning is considered to have come to prominence early in the last century, although it is thought that the notion of learning through life goes back to the time of Plato (http://www.infed.org/lifelonglearning/b-life.htm; accessed 10 September 2012). Lifelong learning is to be distinguished from lifelong education. Education essentially comprises activities normally planned by an education provider, whereas learning is viewed as a cognitive process internal to the learner. Learning occurs through both incidental learning experienced by the learner and by the learner engaging with planned educational experiences, thus through both informal and formal learning opportunities. Lifelong learning is said to foster the continuous improvement of knowledge and skills for personal fulfilment as well as for employment. Often, lifelong learning entails the learner drawing on a mixture of educational programmes and informal learning to develop both capability and potential for managing all aspects of life, including formal employment as desired.

Lifelong learning has been variously defined. One of the more neutral definitions comes from the European Commission. It states that lifelong learning is:

> all learning activity undertaken throughout life, with the aim of improving knowledge, skills and competence, within a personal, civic, social and/or employment-related perspective (European Commission, 2001, p. 9).

This definition embraces all learning, both formal and informal, that occurs from birth to old age and is not specific to learning for or in employment. There are many stages of learning throughout life. Initially, we use innate senses to set us on the road to survival and development, but very early on in our existence, our efforts become increasingly more focused in order to meet personal needs and goals. These needs and goals change over time and our learning capacity extends to cope with the changing demands of work and family life. Informal learning at home and compulsory formal education in school provide us with the grounding for future life and, for many people, the academic qualifications that will form the entry requirements for more specialised education and training. According to Brownhill (2001, p. 73), education and learning are transformational, 'developing an individual's capacity to be a rational autonomous person who respects others ... this is achieved mainly by the process of learning and self-reflection on that learning'. Lifelong learning thus supports us through all stages of life. It underpins the self-fulfilment of each person and not just the requirements of competent performance in a professional role.

The attributes and qualities of the lifelong learner have been researched (Candy, 2000) and are perceived to be as follows:

- An enquiring mind
- 'Helicopter vision'
- Information literacy
- A sense of personal agency
- A repertoire of learning skills
- Interpersonal skills and group membership

However, these attributes are more likely to be recognised within a formal academic environment rather than through working relationships within informal settings. Individuals may still possess these skills even if they go unrecognised. An enquiring mind may lead naturally to personal development through learning from experiences. Those with a sense of personal agency will take steps to engage with new projects and new ventures. They will gather information and use problem-solving skills to develop their capacity to progress in their endeavours. People who value learning will do so for self-fulfilment often without recognising that they are also developing themselves as autonomous lifelong learners. For example, many people in retirement continue learning for self-fulfilment. As far as learning capacity is concerned, those who can draw on a variety of personal learning strategies will benefit most from different learning experiences. Working with others offers opportunity to engage in meaningful conversations and gain different perspectives on new experiences. Every new experience helps build capability for use in later situations.

Lifelong learning is thus wider than making an effort to maintain competence to practise in the professional role. It supports career development and other significant life changes. Lifelong learning thus spans a wide range of education and training initiatives and informal learning opportunities to promote the development of new knowledge and skills, flexibility, creativity, adaptability, preparedness for career and lifestyle change and self-fulfilment at any time of life. Changes may also embrace time out of paid employment, for example maternity leave or the resumption of a career after a career break. They may include changes following redundancy or progression into retirement. Lifelong learning experiences can help make a success of these transitions. A commitment to lifelong learning and CPD can help individuals to counteract the impact of change as well as prepare them for new roles within or beyond a professional career.

Employability

A professional career commences with an education that prepares the individual for a chosen profession or role in employment. Employability denotes a person's capability of being employed in a job (van der Heijden, 2002) and is increasingly used as a measure of success by universities, colleges and other education and training institutions. These institutions are expected to ensure not only that graduates have the specialist skills for their chosen trade or profession but also that they are accomplished in key skills that will help them gain and maintain employment. Key skills are commonly perceived as:

- communication skills;
- teamwork;
- skills of analysis;
- problem-solving skills and creativity;
- enterprise and self-management skills;
- ability to work with technology.

Graduates should also have the incentive for lifelong learning. Education establishments thus are expected to help further develop the skills that underpin lifelong learning. Cheetham and Chivers (1999) initially referred to a selection of these skills as the metacompetencies of competent performance recognised as common across all professions. They went on to define four areas of competence that would vary from profession to profession, namely (1) knowledge/cognitive competence, (2) functional competence, (3) personal behavioural competence and (4) values and ethical competence. A good grounding in the competence requirements of the chosen profession and well-developed employability skills should help secure the new graduate a job. Research has indicated that transition to another job depends more on the possession of a wide range of professional skills and the capability to adjust flexibly to changing circumstances (van der Heijden, 2002). A focus on developing professional expertise is thus important for career mobility. Those with career aspirations need to ensure not only that they remain fit to practise but also that they develop their professional expertise beyond the level of initial competence to practise. Employability is thus a phenomenon that draws on lifelong learning to show the ongoing development and application of key skills in more challenging areas of practice.

The professional career

Definitions of career have changed over time. Arthur et al. (1989) adopted the definition of career as 'the evolving sequence of a person's work experiences over time' (p. 8). This definition provided a 'moving perspective' that the authors considered important, and that acknowledged personal growth and changes over time, and the relationship between a person and a changing society. In 2002, Hall noted changes that had taken place, particularly in relation to organisational change as workplaces grew, merged, downsized and otherwise reinvented themselves, impacting significantly on the workforce. The new term *protean career* (Hall, 2002) came to suggest a greater emphasis on the needs of the person rather than the organisation and an acknowledgement that change of employment over time was becoming the norm. Changes in career direction became acceptable practice, offering opportunities for individuals to seek a greater sense of meaning and purpose in their working life. Work–life balance also gained momentum and came to have a bearing on employment decisions. Part-time employment became the choice of some employees who just wanted greater freedom in their life to pursue other interests beyond work. Generally speaking, however, opportunity to create personal security in work came from the development of skills and an ability to learn rather than from reliance on organisational need. A belief in one's own talents and capacity would allow for more risk-taking. Any uncertainty about jobs drives the need for lifelong learning. Practitioners must take responsibility regularly to review their situation individually, with a mentor or through work appraisal, and consider their longer term future. Relevant personal and professional development opportunities can then be planned. These matters are further addressed in later chapters.

Portfolio careers

Handy (1990) coined the phrase 'portfolio people', denoting those people who had a flexible approach to using their time productively. Just as Arthur et al. (1989) viewed a career as a sequence of jobs, Handy saw the merits of individuals having a variety of employment options, that is, a portfolio of different types of work that could be undertaken simultaneously. Some employment might be paid work and some might be unpaid. For example, undertaking further study or engaging in creative activity or voluntary work might not necessarily contribute to income generation. These might be elective activities that meet a different need and offer personal fulfilment. Some activities, such as gaining an educational qualification, may provide the groundwork for generating income in a different career at a later date. The political context of work can, from time to time, mean that employment is hard to find. Even those working in health or social care environments may not be immune from redundancy if new policies demand reorganisation or where financial savings must be made by the employing organisation. Professionals finding themselves without employment will need to review their options for future employment and the most productive way in which their unique talents may be used. Working flexibly in different paid and/or unpaid occupations may be the best option at the time, rather than one of choice. Some people may not be able to afford to pursue a portfolio of activities as a full-time wage may be important. For others, particularly health care professionals, a portfolio of different types of part-time paid employment may offer much needed financial reward and also enhance job satisfaction. For example, part-time employment in a health or social care organisation and part-time private practice might bring a full-time income. As Handy (1990, p. 214) remarked, 'The redefinition of work in modern society is changing the way we look at our lives and at our priorities.' Any changes to employment in services governed by politics are unpredictable. Strategies for lifelong learning must have their place on the agenda of any health and social care professional working in such organisations. Not only can lifelong learning experiences help transform jobs into exciting careers as they inform the development of new practices and bring benefits for employers, but they can also help prepare professionals for new challenges and opportunities that economic or political changes might bring.

In an uncertain financial climate, planning for a future in retirement is even more important. An ageing population has meant that some governments have increasing expectations that individuals work well into their 60s and possibly their 70s before they are eligible for a pension and that they plan for their retirement. The nature of employment may well change as we get older and a portfolio approach to using time productively in different ways may well assist the transition that inevitably must be made. The portfolio career enables individuals to maintain control of their working life, to plan for and adjust to different stages of their life, to engage in different types of activities that bring different kinds of pleasures and rewards and to manage all the transitions that might be expected for a productive life and retirement.

Given the many changes in the environment and the world of work, in individuals' expectations of a career and in relation to the ways in which individuals may choose to spend their time, it is not surprising that other definitions of 'career' have been coined. In a review of the term 'career', Hall (2002) suggested that it had variously been seen as follows:

- Advancement, that is upward mobility of a person within an organisation.
- A career, that is advancement within a profession as a career.
- A lifelong series of jobs irrespective of the type of occupation or direction of movement.
- A lifelong sequence of role-related experiences that includes paid and unpaid roles.

Hall acknowledged a shift towards focusing on the process of a career and increasingly on a person's right to make choices about employment opportunities. In this respect, values and attitudes come into play. The definition that emerged for Hall was that a career is 'the individually perceived sequence of attitudes and behaviours associated with work-related experiences and activities over the span of the person's life' (Hall, 2002, p. 12).

Thus, work meets numerous personal needs, not just physiological and safety needs but also affiliation, achievement and self-actualisation. However, in order to do this, it is up to individuals to take responsibility for decisions associated with work and other roles. Some decisions may require forward planning and some may demand risk-taking. The choice rests with the individual who is ultimately viewed as an active agent in making choices regarding their career and their career development. A career can go through different stages throughout life as personal circumstances and values change and also as the external environment changes (Woodd, 2000). For this reason, Woodd advocated the need for individuals to continuously review and update plans for career development. Meeting the CPD requirements of the regulatory body will enable professionals to keep practising, but will not necessarily ensure employment. Lifelong learning strategies that enable individuals to develop and grow place them in a stronger position for ongoing employment or for venturing into self-employment.

Ethics and quality of care delivery

CPD has so far been considered as a regulatory requirement that health and social care professionals keep up to date with their practice. Each professional may also be subject to a code of ethics set out by their professional body. Both professional and regulatory bodies tend to have standards or statements that reflect their requirements with regard to professionals' ethical behaviour and practice, placing the responsibility firmly with the individual to act in accordance with these expectations. Employing organisations also expect health and social care professionals to continue to maintain and develop their competence to practise so as to offer efficient and effective service delivery and, wherever possible, quality improvement in practice. Evidence-based practice or minimally evidence-informed practice is strongly encouraged. This places a clear responsibility on each professional to keep up to date with best practice that is informed by research so as to be able to practise ethically and knowledgably. Whilst health and social care services will have a vested interest in encouraging and supporting CPD and in developing expertise in practice, the financial burden for professional development may well rest with the individual. Any organisational support will be welcome, but where organisations are working with financial constraints, the funds to support professional development may not be forthcoming. Some employers tend to have only a minimal interest in employees' development beyond the essential legal requirements of health and safety. Therefore, each professional must take responsibility for planning and participating in development activities so as to at least meet the expected standards. As will be shown in later chapters, not all professional development activities need be costly. A wide range of development activities can be undertaken freely in the workplace or otherwise in association with work-related activities and provide significant opportunities for learning and for the enhancement of practice.

Competence to practise

An exploration of literature leads to the conclusion that 'competence to practise' is a difficult concept to define. Eraut (1994, p. 117) spoke of qualification as being 'a rite of passage into the professional world', 'the climax of rule-guided learning' (p. 125). The qualification confers a social status on individuals and indicates to the general public that those qualified are competent to practise. Barnett (1994) further suggested that competence denoted that an individual could perform tasks to an expected standard. However, he also acknowledged that such a statement was simplistic. He observed that we lived in a changing society, so today's competence might not be suited to tomorrow's client needs and, therefore, calling into question the state of competence beyond the point of qualification. Eraut (2003, p. 1) even called it an 'unproved assumption' that a professional's performance at the point of qualification met the standards for competence, but acknowledged that the assumption was historical and that it was the qualification that became the requirement for a legal license to practise. Obtaining a qualification was only the first step towards continuing learning (Haines, 1997). Gonczi (1999, p. 184) helped clarify some of these assumptions by stating that competence standards developed for any given occupation represented 'the best attempts of a representative group of stakeholders to state the attributes needed to perform the major tasks in the occupation at a particular point in time'. He suggested that they were, however, general attributes for possible contexts of practice but had to evolve as new situations were encountered. This reinforced Barnett's view that competence had to change with social change. Eraut (2003) later suggested that definitions of competence might be divided into those that were individually situated (perceived as attributes of the individual) and those that were socially situated (perceived as situated at the interface between the individual and the society served). He concluded that the latter statement better reflected notions of competence. Griffin and Brownhill (2001) went further to suggest that competence was more than just about reaching a standard, it was embedded in a professional ideology that included a duty to maintain competence at a high level by careful practice and by keeping up to date with developments in the profession. Autonomous professionals thus were expected to have a lifelong commitment to maintaining levels of excellence in practice, arguably more than standard competence. Thus, with qualification and professional status comes the associated responsibility for ensuring continuing competence to practise in a changing world (Alsop, 2001).

The earlier book (Alsop, 2000) focused quite considerably on what constituted competence to practise and hypothesised on how the new regulatory body for UK allied health professionals (the incoming Health Professions Council – HPC) might judge competence, incompetence and lack of competence. As it happens now, competence is not a word that is strongly reflected in the HPC or Health and Care Professions Council (HCPC) literature. The HCPC is more concerned with fitness to practise and that registrants meet its current Standards of Proficiency, Standards of Education, Standards of Conduct, Performance and Ethics and Standards of Continuing Professional Development. The regulatory body is, however, still concerned with how professionals continue their development in the light of changing circumstances. Competence has to be considered as both general and context specific and therefore not static. So, competence in one situation may not be transferable to another. As changes occur in the external environment, practice has to change accordingly, calling 'competence' or 'fitness to practise' into question. Judgements also have to be made about the competence of experts, as opposed to those recently qualified, who will have been judged against the original HPC standards.

The notion of competence to practise thus leads us to consider what professional practice is all about, especially for the health and social care professions. Maintaining competence in an ever-changing world of practice is clearly a responsibility of all professionals. Autonomous professionals should recognise this responsibility and should strive continually to enhance their knowledge and understanding of practice on a daily basis through everyday practice and then periodically through more focused learning opportunities as a contribution to lifelong learning. Higgs and Titchen (2001) explored some of the dimensions of professional practice and claimed that it was people centred, context relevant, authentic and wise. A wise practitioner brings a higher level of knowledge to practice; a capacity to see the bigger picture and meaningful, creative possibilities rather than just solutions. Wise practice embraces the notion of transformation, particularly in relation to transforming practice through careful evaluation of practice and through research initiatives. Accountability also features strongly. Decisions and actions taken by professionals can significantly affect the lives of clients, so maintaining up-to-date professional knowledge is critical to the professional judgements that have to be made, and for which individual professionals are accountable (Ewing & Smith, 2001). Competence to practise is thus the starting point recognised in the attainment of the basic professional qualification. CPD is not only a requirement of continuing registration with a regulatory body but also a fundamental responsibility of a professional to ensure a high level of expertise for serving the needs of clients in the current climate of health and social care delivery.

Continuing professional development

Various definitions of CPD can be found in the literature, but for this book, it is important to consider definitions to which professionals working in health and social care can relate. In the earlier edition of this book, the definition used was as follows:

> Continuing professional development (CPD) is a term commonly used to denote the process of the on-going education and development of health care professionals, from initial qualifying education and for the duration of professional life, in order to maintain competence to practise and increase professional proficiency and expertise (Alsop, 2000, p. 1).

A further definition that has particular relevance to members of the Chartered Institute of Personnel Development (CIPD) is also useful for health and social care professionals:

> Continuing professional development (CPD) is a process by which individuals take control of their own learning and development, by engaging in an on-going process of reflection and action (Megginson & Whitaker, 2007, p. 3).

The combination of messages in these two definitions probably provides a comprehensive view of CPD that places the responsibility firmly with the individual. The individual must:

- recognise that CPD is necessary and the value of undertaking it;
- take control of the process;
- select, initiate, plan and complete relevant learning activities;
- reflect on the process and identify the new learning that has been experienced;
- maintain a record of that learning and its relevance to practice in an appropriate format so that it can be made available to those authorised to review it.

Any health or social care practitioner registered with a regulatory body must additionally meet the specific requirements of that body, and these vary considerably across continents. Each regulatory body across the world has its own definition, standards and requirements of those expected to maintain their competence to practise through continuous learning. Registrants should thus acquaint themselves with the specific requirements of their regulatory body.

The UK HPC (now the HCPC), for example, defined CPD as follows:

> A range of learning activities through which health professionals maintain and develop throughout their career to ensure that they retain their capacity to practise safely, effectively and legally within their evolving scope of practice (HPC, 2010, p. 6).

This definition has a specific remit to support regulated professionals in meeting their obligation to practise safely, legally and ethically, and the regulatory body's ultimate remit to protect the public. One further definition is that coined in a joint statement on CPD for health and social care practitioners:

> [CPD] is fundamental to the development of all health and social care practitioners, and is the mechanism through which high quality patient and client care is identified, maintained and developed (RCN, 2007, p. 2).

This statement is useful as not only it clarifies that CPD focuses on an outcome of high-quality patient and client care but the document also specifies that these development activities exclude those that are otherwise required by law, for example manual handling training. Furthermore, it suggests that a minimum 6 days per year should be granted by employers to facilitate this learning activity.

CPD is unquestionably a professional responsibility. However, it also brings personal gains. Undertaking CPD is about recognising the duty of care and taking pride in all aspects of work with and for service users; it is about enhancing personal skills and confidence and thus professional capability; it is about investing in oneself as well as developing the knowledge and skills required by employers. Any investment in CPD could bring just rewards especially at times when competition for jobs is strong. CPD ultimately adds interest to the job and becomes the building blocks on which a professional career is founded. Autonomous professionals should not wait for CPD opportunities to be offered but should actively seek out opportunities that support their ambitions and career goals. CPD does not have to be expensive nor depend on funding from employers. This book offers many suggestions for CPD activities that can be pursued with little or no cost. Funding may, however, be available for CPD that will clearly enhance service provision or bring efficiency savings. A case for funding would normally have to be made, and even if successful, full funding may not be forthcoming. Applicants need to be prepared to supplement any financial grant they receive in order to engage in the selected CPD activity. However, this still becomes an investment for the future.

Summary

This chapter has considered the value of lifelong learning for personal and career development throughout life. Lifelong learning has a wide remit assisting an individual to become self-fulfilled and participate in education, work or leisure pursuits throughout life. The development of general skills for employment forms an essential feature of all graduate education. For health and social care professionals, formal university education has to meet the specific requirements of regulatory and professional bodies, addressing features of competence and fitness to practise in the chosen profession. Contemporary definitions of a career have been discussed and applied to careers in health and social care. Personal and professional development has been shown to be essential for the maintenance of high-quality care. Definitions of continuing professional development (CPD) have set the scene for wider discussions on the CPD expectations of regulatory bodies and the audit process. CPD is the term that tends to be used by regulatory bodies as a legal requirement for continuing registration.

References

Alsop A (2000) *Continuing Professional Development: A Guide for Therapists*. Blackwell Science, Oxford.

Alsop A (2001) Competence unfurled: developing portfolio practice. *Occupational Therapy International*, **8** (2), 126–131.

Arthur MB, Hall DT & Lawrence BS (1989) Generating new directions in career theory: the case for a transdisciplinary approach. In: *Handbook of Career Theory* (eds MB Arthur, DT Hall & BS Lawrence), pp. 7–25. Cambridge University Press, Cambridge.

Barnett R (1994) *The Limits of Competence*. Society for Research into Higher Education and Open University Press, Buckingham.

Brownhill B (2001) Lifelong learning. In: *The Age of Learning Education and the Knowledge Society* (ed. P Jarvis), pp. 69–79. Kogan Page, London.

Candy PC (2000) Reaffirming a proud tradition: universities and lifelong learning. *Active Learning in Higher Education*, **1** (2), 101–125.

Cheetham G & Chivers G (1999) Professional competence harmonizing reflective practitioner and competence-based approaches. In: *Developing the Capable Practitioner, Professional Capability through Higher Education* (eds D O'Reilly, L Cunningham &S Lester), pp. 215–228. Kogan Page, London.

Eraut M (1994) *Developing Professional Knowledge and Competence*. Falmer Press, London.

Eraut M (2003) Editorial. *Learning in Health and Social Care*, **2** (1), 1–5.

European Commission (2001) *Making a European Area of Lifelong Learning a Reality*. www.bologna-berlin2003.de/pdf/mitteilungeng.pdf (accessed 23 October 2012).

Ewing R & Smith D (2001) Becoming in professional practice: an exemplar. In: *Professional Practice in Health, Education and the Creative Arts* (eds J Higgs & A Titchen), pp. 175–184. Blackwell Science, Oxford.

Gonczi A (1999) Competency-based learning: a dubious past – an assured future? In: *Understanding Learning at Work* (eds D Boud & J Garrick), pp. 180–195. Routledge, London.

Griffin C & Brownhill B (2001) The learning society. In: *The Age of Learning: Education and the Knowledge Society* (ed. P Jarvis), pp. 55–68. Kogan Page, London.

Haines P (1997) Professionalization through CPD: is it realistic for achieving our goals? *British Journal of Therapy and Rehabilitation*, **4**, 428–447.

Hall DT (2002) *Careers In and Out of Organizations*. Sage Publications, Thousand Oaks, CA.

Handy C (1990) *Inside Organizations: 21 Ideas for Managers*. BBC Books, London.

Higgs J & Titchen A (eds) (2001) Framing professional practice: knowing and doing in context. In: *Professional Practice in Health, Education and the Creative Arts*, pp. 3–15. Blackwell Science, Oxford.

HPC (2010) *CPD and Your Registration*. Health Professions Council, London.

Megginson D & Whitaker V (2007) *Continuing Professional Development*, 2nd edn. Chartered Institute of Personnel Management, London.

RCN (2007) *Joint Statement of Continuing Professional Development for Health and Social Care Practitioners*. Royal College of Nursing, London.

Van der Heijden B (2002) Pre-requisites to guarantee life-long employability. *Personnel Review*, **31** (1), 44–61.

Woodd M (2000) The psychology of career theory – a new perspective? *Career Development International*, **5** (6), 273–278.

Chapter 2

Regulation of allied health and social care professionals

This chapter addresses:

1. the responsibilities of regulated health and social care professionals to maintain records of continuing professional development (CPD) activity;
2. the rationale for CPD in relation to career development;
3. the audit process of the Health and Care Professions Council (HCPC).

Introduction

Many health and social care professionals, both across the United Kingdom and in other countries, are regulated by law. The designated regulatory body of each state, province or country (as applicable) sets out the standards and other expectations for each registered professional to ensure protection of the public. Public protection is the primary remit of all bodies regulating health and social care professionals in their practice. Practitioners who meet the standards and requirements of the regulatory body are registered, but then they have ongoing responsibilities with regard to professional development in order to remain on the register and continue to be eligible to practise in their chosen profession. Continuing professional development (CPD) is one requirement of each registrant to ensure that practice remains up to date and continues to be carried out ethically, legally and with due regard for client safety.

In some countries, students of the health care professions, assistants and support workers employed in health and social care settings must also be registered. They are normally subject to education, training and development requirements that are specific to their role. Other countries such as the United Kingdom currently only register those who have become qualified for their profession by attending a formal university programme and meeting the set education and proficiency standards of the established regulatory body. Registration is normally not transferable from one regulatory body to another, so anyone wishing to move to practise in another country,

Continuing Professional Development in Health and Social Care: Strategies for Lifelong Learning, Second Edition. Auldeen Alsop.
© 2013 John Wiley & Sons, Ltd. Published 2013 by John Wiley & Sons, Ltd.

state or province, for instance, will need to apply to, and meet the requirements of, the new regulatory body. This may mean undertaking further study, taking an examination and/or completing other practice requirements, as required by the new regulator. Evidence may also be required of the applicant having kept up to date with practice through CPD.

This chapter explores the general expectations of regulatory bodies drawing mainly, but not exclusively, on the model of the UK Health and Care Professions Council (HCPC) to provide examples of systems in use. Generally, registered health and care professionals must periodically show evidence of CPD for continued registration with their regulatory body. There are similar expectations from professionals in countries such as Canada, the United States, Australia, New Zealand and South Africa, but each country, and sometimes each state or province, has specific expectations and requirements that must be followed by individual registrants. Current details of these expectations, including those of the UK HCPC, can be found on the relevant website. This chapter offers a guide to the types of responsibilities and requirements of the registrant and to the process of meeting those requirements.

The UK Health and Care Professions Council

This council is currently responsible for registering the following allied health and care professionals:

- Art therapists
- Biomedical scientists
- Chiropodists/podiatrists
- Clinical scientists
- Dieticians
- Hearing aid dispensers
- Occupational therapists
- Operating department practitioners
- Orthoptists
- Paramedics
- Physiotherapists
- Practitioner psychologists
- Prosthetists/orthotists
- Radiographers
- Social workers
- Speech and language therapists

Regulatory bodies in other countries each have their own list of professions whose practitioners must register in order to practise in their profession. There are variations across the world. Some of the above professions may be excluded whilst others not listed above are included in a national register. Some professions may be very newly recognised as registrants with a regulatory body. Many countries do not yet have systems in place for regulation of the professions. Nevertheless, even if not registered, all health and social care professionals are required to practise ethically and maintain competence in their professional role, as often laid down in the profession's relevant Code of Ethics and Professional Conduct.

In the United Kingdom, all qualified practitioners in the above professions are required to register and, as a responsibility of registration, must demonstrate that they engage in CPD activities in order to keep themselves up to date with practice. Registrants must keep a record of these activities and if they are selected for audit of their CPD activity, they must produce the record within an allocated time and forward it to the HCPC to be assessed by appointed assessors. More detail is given later about the process.

Specific requirements of registrants regarding their CPD

Currently, in the United Kingdom, a registrant must:

1. maintain a continuous, up-to-date and accurate record of their CPD activities;
2. demonstrate that their CPD activities are a mixture of learning activities relevant to current or future practice;
3. seek to ensure that their CPD has contributed to the quality of their practice and service delivery;
4. seek to ensure that their CPD benefits the service user;
5. upon request, present a written profile (which must be their own work and supported by evidence) explaining how they have met the standards for CPD.
       Source: Health Professions Council (HPC) Information (for registrants), CPD and your registration (HPC, 2010, p. 6).

Other countries use different systems for logging CPD activity. Some use a points system. The regulatory body lays down the total number of points that each registrant must collect from CPD activity within a given timeframe. CPD providers can apply to have their activity rated for points. Registrants then tot up the points accumulated through attendance at, and participation in, a number of points-rated activities. The list of activities, totalling the required number of points and fulfilling any other specific requirements with regard to topics addressed, is submitted to the regulatory body on demand, if selected for audit. For example, currently in South Africa, professionals must complete CPD activities to a total value of 30 points each year, including activities within specified categories, such as ethics, human rights and medical law. Assistants must achieve 15 points in the same way (www.hpcsa.co.za; accessed 30 January 2012).

Expectations of the practitioner

It is the duty of each registrant to remain competent to practise in his or her profession. However, it has to be argued that CPD should not just be a requirement of registration, it should be at the heart of each professional's practice to enable that person to grow and fulfil his or her potential at all stages of a professional career. This marks out CPD as a long-term process rather than an end product or merely a target for ongoing registration. The CPD requirement applies equally to those working in clinical practice, management, education or research. The nature of CPD may have a slightly different bias, dependent on the focus of work, but still has the aim of improving practice. So if it is accepted that CPD is a long-term process spanning the full period of a professional's career, then there is a need to pay attention to the process throughout all the changes in employment and over the spectrum of a career. CPD is thus seen as an individual professional's responsibility. It can be planned to facilitate professional growth or it can emerge through different experiences in professional life. These experiences have to be revisited, reviewed systematically and then translated, through reflection and evaluation, into learning. For the purpose of demonstrating ongoing competence to the HCPC, the benefits to the service user and to the individual registrant of the professional's new learning must be made explicit.

Initial pre-registration education and continuing professional development

Of those who choose employment in the health or social care system, some may find work as assistants or support workers and have school-leaving qualifications only to their credit. However, even at this level some countries such as the United States have expectations that individuals additionally gain specific, recognised qualifications at certificate level in order to practise. Those wishing to go on to gain a professional qualification will normally undertake a university course and emerge with a bachelor's degree, Master's degree or professional doctorate that is recognised and approved by the regulatory body. Irrespective of the academic level, this formal award will be the basic professional qualification. Further formal or informal learning will still be required as an ongoing commitment to professional and career development.

Formal learning in support of a professional's career starts during initial pre-registration education. Students of the professions are guided through their programme so as ultimately to attain the required knowledge, skills, aptitudes and standards to allow them to apply for registration. In some countries, once an appropriate professional diploma or degree has been awarded, an additional examination must be passed for registration purposes. The initial learning process includes developing and using skills of reflection and evaluation. The identification of new learning from experiences and ways of documenting the learning and its relevance to practice are skills that must also be acquired. Opportunities for developing these attributes are built into pre-registration programmes so that students become conversant with the notion of lifelong learning, skills and activities associated with learning and CPD prior to qualification. The continuity of the process of learning established prior to professional education, refined during the qualifying programme and progressing into professional practice is thus reinforced. Pre-registration education also promotes the constant refinement of learning skills so that activities associated with undertaking and recording CPD become well rehearsed. These skills and activities are discussed more fully in later chapters.

Beyond initial professional education

It has to be noted that there is a distinct difference between the learning experiences in initial professional education and those associated with continuing professional education and development. Skills of competent performance are initially developed and assessed through a defined professional pre-registration programme that allows for the systematic attainment, development and application of knowledge and skills associated with practice. All students of a profession follow a prescribed curriculum to meet standards that lead to the right to apply for registration with a regulatory body. CPD, on the other hand, has to be self-initiated and self-directed. Learning activities are normally tailored specifically to meet individual needs and may take many forms. Learning must be planned and negotiated personally rather than being structured and assessed by others. Judgements about competence formerly undertaken by other people now have to be built into professional practice in the form of self-evaluation of personal performance.

A professional's ability to judge and evaluate his or her own performance is necessary so as to be able to learn from practice. However, this is a difficult task and requires well-developed skills of reflection and critical evaluation of personal performance. Making the shift from engaging in a structured learning programme that others assess, to devising and implementing a personal learning strategy that is self-assessed can be difficult. Managing a workload, managing learning and integrating learning systematically into professional life is not easy. It takes time, self-discipline and good personal organisation. In order to commit to developing themselves professionally, practitioners have to see the potential benefits and then develop the skills to ensure that learning and professional development become integral to practice and not just an adjunct to it. CPD will only be of real benefit if the learning takes place as a voluntary activity, as part of a process of lifelong learning and as part of a personal commitment to self-development. Whilst CPD might be a requirement of continued registration, it really is more than that. CPD activity needs to be a valued and meaningful aspect of professional practice. Initially, professional development is integral to learning that takes place within a professional qualifying programme. CPD is an extended part of practice that has an additional time commitment to allow for reflection on practice and the identification of new learning.

Some of the benefits of CPD can thus be listed as follows:

- Ethically continuing to offer best practice to service users.
- Encouraging a higher standard of personal professional performance.
- Demonstrating a commitment to best practice.
- Demonstrating a professional commitment to service users.
- Demonstrating a commitment to current and future employers.
- Providing increased job scope and job satisfaction.

- Providing the means to anticipate, plan and prepare for change.
- Enhancing professional knowledge, skills and status.
- Promoting awareness of new developments and concepts.
- Expanding areas of personal expertise.
- Improving personal efficiency.
- Providing a framework for making informed decisions about future professional activity.
- Improving career prospects and the ability to assume new roles.
- Providing opportunity to develop networks of people with similar skills and interests.

Any one of these reasons could provide sufficient grounds for contemplating and engaging in CPD irrespective of the requirements associated with registration. Changes in direction from practice into management, education or research can also be contemplated.

Planned CPD activity is not the only means of learning. Taking advantage of unplanned scenarios or situations that offer new experiences and thus new learning is always valuable. Critical reflection on these unexpected experiences and follow-up by reference to literature or through communication with other relevant people will provide new insights on practice that can be logged as learning experiences. Further guidance on developing and using these skills is addressed later in the book.

CPD and career enhancement

Health and social care professionals have an obligation to remain fit to practise in their chosen profession, but beyond that they should take responsibility for both shaping change (Barnett, 1994) and for making a personal contribution to the growth of their profession. They should do this by enhancing knowledge and understanding, and placing it in the public domain (Barnett, 1997), potentially through scholarly or other professional activity. This would suggest that individual practitioners should show a commitment to their profession as well as to themselves and commit to learning throughout professional life. Lifelong learning goes even beyond that. The era of having a job for life, even within a chosen profession, has long passed. The external environment and contexts of work are fast changing and the situation requires flexible people who have developed the capacity to fulfil different roles and can adapt quickly and efficiently to changing circumstances. Practitioners must now anticipate the need to work in news ways, change direction and shift the emphasis in respect of their professional responsibilities as the environment changes. Political, economic, sociological and technical changes can all influence the way in which health and social care is delivered. Philosophical shifts such as the developing emphasis on taking personal responsibility for maintaining health can also impact on the priorities of service provision and thus on ways of working.

Health and social care professionals also need to take stock of their careers from time to time. Some may choose to adapt or respond to environmental changes in different ways, for example by moving into private practice. Some may adopt different roles within their employing organisation in managerial, leadership, advisory, educational or research positions. Others may review their personal circumstances and skills and then make life-changing decisions about their career, and set off in a completely new direction. Whatever the choice, learning and developing the capacity to assume new roles are critical for success. Decisions regarding learning and development are personal, as are the responsibilities for organising and financing any development opportunity and for managing the undertaking in association with other personal commitments. Employing organisations may see advantages in promoting CPD and thus offer to fund, or make a contribution towards funding, professional development. However, the potential benefits of the education to clients may need to be demonstrated in a business case to the employer prior to finance being agreed. Alternatively, other sponsorship may be sought. Essentially, CPD primarily benefits the individual undertaking it as it enhances personal practice. However, services and service users also benefit from that practice; hence, one of the requirements of the HCPC is for those benefits to services and service users to be made explicit in the audit process.

Meeting the requirements of the UK HCPC

One of the purposes of this book is to assist health and social care professionals to address the requirements of their regulatory body with regard to CPD and thus maintain eligibility to be on the relevant register. The first step in meeting the regulatory body requirements is to gain familiarity with its expectations especially if periodic audit of CPD activity is mandatory. It is common for those expectations to be clearly set out in written form and to be sent to each registrant, and also to be available via the official website of the regulatory body. Every registrant must be prepared to fulfil the requirements. In practice, only a small proportion of those registered are normally targeted each year to produce and submit evidence of CPD according to specifications for the official audit. All other registrants are required to certify that they have undertaken CPD activities with a view to maintaining their professional competence. The official website of the UK HCPC is: www.hcpc-uk.org.

The HCPC has its own definition of CPD. CPD is defined as:

> A range of learning activities through which health professionals maintain and develop throughout their career to ensure that they retain their capacity to practise safely, effectively and legally within their evolving scope of practice (HPC, 2010, p. 6).

Whilst this definition of CPD is specific to the UK HCPC, the HCPC is clear that it sees no automatic link between CPD and competence. Competence can be maintained without CPD and CPD does not guarantee competence. The actual link has thus to be made. All registrants are expected to maintain a continuous, up-to-date and accurate record of their CPD activities. These activities must be a mixture of learning activities relevant to current or future practice. The registrant must show how the activities have contributed to the quality of practice and service delivery and ensure that the benefit to service users can be demonstrated. Various CPD activities are acceptable for the audit and it is recognised that those activities may be different depending on the employment of the registrant in a clinical role, management, education or research. It is also important to note that not every aspect of CPD that is undertaken has to be submitted for the audit. The CPD activities should be carefully selected from all those documented in preparation for the audit so as to demonstrate a range of learning initiatives that have positively impacted on the care management of service users.

The HCPC is clear that its standards focus on quality of outcomes, in particular for service users, and not on the number of hours spent engaging in CPD activity. As already noted, some other regulatory bodies require a list of CPD activities that together achieve a target number of points. This is why it is important to be absolutely clear about the CPD requirements of your regulatory body. This also applies to students and support workers in countries where registration of these individuals is the norm.

Registrants may, from time to time, take a break from practising their profession. This may not necessarily mean allowing registration to lapse. CPD activity has to be maintained in these circumstances. Even if registration lapses, it is advisable to continue to maintain a CPD profile whilst taking a break so as to be able to demonstrate ongoing competence should return to practice be desired. Those practitioners wishing to return to practice after a break will need to acquaint themselves with the specific requirements of the regulatory body.

Submissions for CPD audit

The HCPC sets out specifically on its website and in written documentation what has to be submitted for its audit. Each profession is audited separately and only a small number of registrants are randomly selected for audit each time. Those registrants required to submit their CPD activity are advised by post and are given plenty of time to prepare the submission. Written instructions sent to registrants give details of what has to be submitted. It must be recognised by registrants that this is an important process for ongoing registration and failure to comply could ultimately mean that the registrant's name is removed from the register. This is a last resort, but can happen, with the consequence that the professional may not practise again as a registered practitioner until he or she has completed the re-registration process. Timeframes and requirements are strictly observed by the HCPC and so should not be ignored. As with most formal requirements, the HCPC instructions for submitting details of professional development activities should be read carefully and followed explicitly. The submission does not have to be complicated, just thorough in its presentation, which should clearly and succinctly address the given requirements of the audit.

Currently, the HCPC sends out a profile for completion to those registrants selected for audit. The profile has to show how the registrant has met the CPD standards. The profile, with relevant evidence to support it, must be returned to the HCPC for assessment. In brief, there are three parts to the profile[1]:

1. A summary of practice over the previous 2 years (up to 500 words).
2. A statement detailing how the CPD standards have been met, the CPD activities undertaken (which must be a variety of activities) and details of the supporting evidence (up to 1500 words).
3. The evidence of CPD activities undertaken and how they have contributed to improving the quality of practice and benefited service users.

Requirements are always subject to change, so the regulatory body must always be consulted for up-to-date information about the audit process.

The HPC that preceded the HCPC (HPC, 2010) identified from earlier audits a number of practices that should be avoided. Some of these are summarised below.

Registrants should *not*:

- send confidential information, including patient records;
- forget to send a list of CPD activities undertaken during the previous 2 years, as required;
- forget to distinguish between everyday work activities and activities specifically undertaken for CPD;
- list activities without specifying how they contribute to learning;
- refer assessors to an online log of activities rather than completing documentation as required;
- use profession-specific abbreviations excessively;
- send large folders of evidence instead of a few examples carefully selected to illustrate how specific requirements were met.

These and other similar practices suggest that registrants have previously not followed the guidelines outlined by the HCPC. Most specifically, they have not identified for the assessors the specific CPD activities that have been undertaken or have not indicated the way in which the activities contributed to CPD. If the submission is incomplete then assessors will ask for further information. Once all information is submitted and the assessors are satisfied that the standards have been met, the individual will be informed and the registration should continue. Those who initially do not meet the standards may be given more time to submit more information. However, assessors may recommend that registration should end if a registrant ultimately does not meet the standards.

The experience of audit

The key message for those having to submit a profile of their work for assessment is to ensure that the current specific requirements of the regulatory body are understood

---

[1]This information is indicative of the kind of evidence required by the UK regulatory body at the time of going to press. The HCPC should always be consulted about the up-to-date requirements for the audit.

and followed explicitly. Given that the audit process has now been in operation for a few years, a number of people from each profession will have completed the profile. It will always help to talk to anyone who has had to submit their work. In 2009, Melanie Larkin was targeted for audit. Her account (Larkin, 2010) of the experience probably sums up what many audited professionals have felt about the process. The various emotions associated with first receiving the letter and then preparing the documentation are made evident in Larkin's story. Some messages emerge from this account:

- Most people think that, given the small percentage of each profession being targeted each time, it is unlikely to happen to them. It can happen.
- Most professionals have good intentions with regard to keeping an up-to-date CPD portfolio. However, it is easy to allow this to lapse, causing panic should it be needed.
- Reading professional literature and writing reflections of CPD activities can be personally and professionally rewarding, and not just a chore.

Most professional bodies now have guidance available to assist members in this process, so it is worth checking with their website and seeking support.

Summary

A commitment to lifelong learning is a professional responsibility of registered health and social care professionals in order to maintain and develop personal skills as well as to contribute to the growth of the profession. Lifelong learning also assists with career development. Regulation of health and social care professionals also brings specific responsibilities for those on the register. Not only is there an ethical responsibility to keep up to date with practice for public protection by engaging in continuing professional development (CPD), but there is also a requirement to maintain a record of CPD activities should the registrant be called to produce the evidence of CPD in an audit by the regulatory body. Regulatory bodies in different countries work on similar principles but may have significantly different requirements. Transfer of registration between regulatory bodies in different countries is thus not normally permitted. Each registrant must ensure familiarity with the requirements of the relevant regulatory body for CPD when practising or when taking a break from practice.

References

Barnett R (1994) *The Limits of Competence*. Society for Research into Higher Education and Open University Press, Buckingham.
Barnett R (1997) *Higher Education: A Critical Business*. Society for Research into Higher Education and Open University Press, Buckingham.
HPC (2010) *Continuing Professional Development and Your Registration*. Health Professions Council, London.
Larkin M (2010) The HPC audit – it happened to me! *OT News*, **18** (8), 42.

Chapter 3

The professional portfolio

This chapter addresses:

1. definitions and the purpose of compiling professional portfolios and profiles;
2. maintaining records in manual and e-portfolios for career purposes;
3. the regulatory body's continuing professional development (CPD) audit expectations and requirements.

Introduction

Professional portfolios have become popular with health and social care practitioners as a means of collecting and presenting evidence of learning and continuing professional development (CPD). Portfolios have been developed and maintained for use in a variety of situations and, for this reason, may take a variety of forms. It is worth remembering where the word 'portfolio' came from. 'Portfolio' derived from the Latin *portare* meaning 'to carry' and *folium* meaning 'a leaf' and is now commonly defined as a 'collection of papers' such as those put together by an artist to show the range and quality of his or her work and capacity for employment. Professional bodies now commonly use the term portfolio to denote a method that their members can use for keeping records of education, training and learning experiences in which they have engaged. It is recommended that every professional (practising or non-practising) maintains records of learning activity and includes the evidence of that activity for later reference. Although not every learning experience will be documented, learning is, in fact, going on all the time in professional practice. Only selected key activities thus need to be recorded, such as those that demonstrate a particular aspect of professional development and growth. These records can show that any previously identified learning needs have been met and may sometimes demonstrate capacity for promotion. The fact that a portfolio is being updated indicates that it is a dynamic entity responsive to the changing needs of practice and the owner. Redman (1994, p. 42) advised that a portfolio 'is not a historical record of

Continuing Professional Development in Health and Social Care: Strategies for Lifelong Learning, Second Edition. Auldeen Alsop.
© 2013 John Wiley & Sons, Ltd. Published 2013 by John Wiley & Sons, Ltd.

achievement, nor a current profile of competence, but a living, growing collection of evidence that mirrors the growth of its owner, including his or her hopes and plans for the future'.

The term portfolio has actually been defined as:

> a collection of evidence which demonstrates the continuing acquisition of skills, knowledge, attitudes, understanding and achievement. It is both retrospective and prospective as well as reflecting the current stage of development and activity of the individual (Brown, 1992, p. 1).

One of the key words in both observations above is 'evidence'. The fact that evidence is what counts in portfolio composition makes us realise that we actually have to judge what evidence is and discount everything that does not contribute to the evidence. Brown and Knight (1994, p. 82) saw a portfolio not as a heap of everything that came to hand but as a carefully selected range of artefacts that show progression and demonstrate improvement over time. So it is important to discriminate when it comes to choosing what goes in and what stays out of a portfolio.

The term portfolio has purposely been introduced early in this chapter as it could be perceived to have a broader meaning than the term 'profile', another term in common usage. Brown (1992) has helpfully distinguished between the terms portfolio and profile, suggesting that a *profile* is a collection of evidence that is selected from a *portfolio* for a particular purpose and for the attention of a particular audience. Although these descriptions may not be used universally, it could be suggested that a portfolio contains a wider range of references and evidence than a profile. From a portfolio, an informed choice of material can be made to be presented as a profile of the individual for a particular purpose. A profile can have different uses. However, it is a term that is particularly relevant to practising health care professionals in the United Kingdom. Profile is the term currently used by the UK Health and Care Professions Council (HCPC) to indicate the format in which information must be submitted by a registrant to show that he or she continues to meet the HCPC CPD standards (HPC, 2010). The structure and requirements of the profile are set out by the HCPC. A random sample of each profession's registrants is currently audited every 2 years. Current expectations are always available on the HCPC website (www.hcpc-uk.org) and these are sent to each registrant of a named profession who is part of the sample when the audit of that profession's CPD occurs.

Variations of portfolio

It is now generally an expectation of students of the health and social care professions that they develop and maintain a portfolio during their professional qualifying education. Universities tend to introduce students to portfolio construction and use early on in their course so that they become accustomed to the practice of reflecting on their experiences, recording their learning and developing action plans for the future. For some students, portfolio records may even form part of an assessment. A range of creative assessments may also be devised to demonstrate the development of particular knowledge and skills. The portfolio could be the medium through which some assignments are submitted for marking. However, it is important to state that at this stage of a student's professional development the emphasis is on student learning rather than on the creation of a perfect portfolio.

Portfolios may also take a variety of forms. Manual portfolios have been in common usage for some time. They have allowed for record keeping and the storage of key information and evidence of learning. Increasingly, e-portfolios have become the instrument of choice for recording and managing personal information and evidence of CPD. Universities may have their own online scheme or may subscribe to a commercial scheme such as PebblePad for use by students. It is worth considering how both manual and e-portfolios are used.

Manual portfolios

Manual portfolios have tended to comprise a loose-leaf file that is organised by its owner into sections that are personally meaningful and from which information may be drawn selectively for a particular purpose. Not all information in the portfolio will be applicable every time a portfolio is presented. For example, information to fulfil the requirements of an assessment will not be the same as information required to support an application for an interview. Not all information in a portfolio need ever be made public – sections can be kept for personal use only. Selective reflections and observations made for learning purposes that the owner may not wish to share might be a part of this section. Even if the portfolio is well maintained and comprehensive, it is still likely to be too big for any specific task, so selectivity is essential every time the portfolio is used. Information to be extracted from the portfolio will thus be selected according to the need that has to be fulfilled. A carefully constructed filing system and index will allow relevant material to be located quickly.

Although portfolios may commonly be kept for CPD purposes, it is worth noting that they can have different uses, for example:

- Demonstrating learning as a course participant.
- Demonstrating the achievement of learning outcomes for an assessment.
- Providing evidence of experiential learning that may be presented for accreditation.
- Providing evidence of competence to practise.
- Providing evidence of advanced practice.
- Showing evidence of ongoing critical evaluation of practice.
- Showing evidence of academic progress, for example through written feedback from tutors.
- Providing evidence of professional development and continuing competence.
- Demonstrating that specific criteria have been met and readiness for promotion.
- Demonstrating fulfilment of criteria for a new job.
- Demonstrating additional strengths and skills, for example as an educator.
- Demonstrating career development and progression over time.
- Presenting skills and abilities that can be marketed.

It is clear to see that evidence is important and that the material presented for any of these purposes should make a contribution as evidence. E-portfolios can be put to similar use.

E-portfolios

E-portfolios are more difficult to define. Even some of those responsible for designing e-portfolios find it difficult to present a definition. One definition offered by the creators of PebblePad is that an e-portfolio:

> is a purposeful aggregation of digital items – ideas, evidence, reflections, feedback, etc. – which 'presents' a selected audience with evidence of a person's learning and/or ability (http://www.pebblepad.co.uk/; accessed 1 December 2011).

Arguably, the definition is similar to those offered for manual portfolios, which may go some way towards appeasing those who still prefer to use manual systems. The difference between manual and electronic systems is the way in which material is created and held within the system, and the ways in which it can be used. As an e-portfolio, PebblePad allows users to selectively record any abilities, events, plans or thoughts that are personally significant. However, the data can additionally be linked to other data on the system, so acting as a personal repository for material that can be resurrected for different purposes, as required. An additional function of e-learning systems is that they tend to have in-built mechanisms for promoting learning. For example, the learner may be prompted by the system to consider different aspects of their experience in order to make sense of it and learn from it. Processing information in different ways, for example reflecting on, analysing, interpreting, synthesising and presenting material, may help the learner to gain much more from the entry than otherwise thought. This material can be systematically stored and retrieved. The system will also allow the learner to link entries with evidence, for example records of attending courses or other learning events. Of course, anyone with an e-portfolio may additionally have to store physical evidence such as certificates of attendance at an event, although these could be scanned and added into the e-portfolio. E-portfolios have helped to broaden the ways in which evidence of learning can be developed and stored. However, technology is fast changing and it can be expected that even more sophisticated devices than e-portfolios may be used in future. The Chartered Society of Physiotherapy for some time has recommended the use of PebblePad to its members. PebblePad usage may start during qualifying education but will still be available to individuals on graduation and beyond into their professional life. Access to university systems normally ceases on graduation, which could mean building up a portfolio again from scratch. Using PebblePad or other similar commercial system has the advantage of continuity of use as a practitioner enters practice.

Scrapbooking

All types of portfolio permit the owner to be creative. No form of portfolio should inhibit its owner from presenting material that has inspired learning. There should be no restrictions; the portfolio should serve as the medium for displaying artefacts to the best advantage. The use of scrapbooking enables pictures, photographs, sketches, diagrams, mind maps and other meaningful artefacts to be used as an entry in the portfolio and arranged in such a way as to represent, sometimes symbolically, things that have inspired learning or represent future aspirations. Many of these assets can be accommodated in a manual portfolio. Large items, those that are multi-dimensional and those that have complex compositions, may be better portrayed using scanning processes and e-portfolios. Electronic devices allow for great flexibility in portraying ideas, maximising creativity and offering them to audiences far and wide. Scrapbooking in a manual form may better present artefacts that rely on senses such as touch.

Journaling and creative writing

Different people have different strengths and choose to record their thoughts, ideas, inspirations and aide-mémoires in different ways. Some use pictures, photographs or drawings, others prefer stories or even poems. Journals may be preferred by those who use the written word to portray their learning and their ideas. Some writing could be classed as personal and used for developing new insights into particularly difficult situations. Allowing thoughts to come freely during the writing phase could allow emotions, frustrations and regrets to be explored, balanced wherever possible with pleasurable activities and insights about personal effectiveness and ways for-ward in life. Re-reading what has been written could further one's knowledge and understanding of the impact of certain experiences and lead to new insights. It may be that the original writing always remains in that 'personal and private' section of the portfolio and that a short summary of learning is captured as a synopsis of the original but for wider use. Some people choose to work through metaphors or a third person in a story or poem. It really does not matter provided that the activity serves to enhance knowledge and experience. The spontaneous creativity that is set down during journaling may have little meaning to others. Some thought needs to be given to ways of presenting to others the essence of the material as learning or as meaningful observations.

Profiles

Portfolios, manual or electronic, offer the capacity to store records of experiences that have led to learning. As mentioned earlier in this chapter, the UK HCPC uses the term profile as the format in which information about CPD activity and its effects are to be presented for audit. Only a very small percentage of health professionals are targeted annually for audit; but, whilst the HCPC is clear that evidence of CPD activity may be collected in any way, as chosen by the individual, the evidence of meeting HCPC standards that is submitted to the HCPC must be in a particular format known as a 'profile'. The HCPC currently does not accept profiles or evidence electronically, so the material that is used to demonstrate CPD and professional growth will be drawn from either manual or electronic files and presented in written format. The professional has, however, only to provide evidence of CPD for the 2 years prior to the audit. CPD activity that has taken place before that is not normally required. All registrants should be aware of what the HCPC audit entails (www.hcpc-uk.org) and note any changes to requirements as they are introduced. These may impact on the choice of method of keeping and managing a portfolio.

The student portfolio

Students of the health and social care professions will normally have been introduced to portfolios early in their educational programme and will have been expected to update it throughout their period of learning. As indicated earlier, the main focus of the portfolio in the university will be to help maximise learning. Students may have had a particular format of portfolio recommended to them or may have been required to use, for example, a specific electronic learning tool as part of their course. Once the student leaves the university as a graduate, he or she then has to make decisions about how to continue recording learning activity for the future. In the United Kingdom, a new graduate will not immediately be part of the HCPC audit process. Nevertheless, their CPD activity and learning will need to be recorded for the future. Other countries, especially those where students are registered, may have different expectations.

The first use of a portfolio on, or just before, graduation may well be at the job interview. It is now common practice for job applicants to take a portfolio to interview, but mindful of earlier comments in this chapter, the graduate should create a profile of him or herself drawing on relevant material from the portfolio, as applicable to the job. Up to this stage, the portfolio will largely be a learning portfolio that includes details of academic and practice experiences and successes, and any additional awards given by the university. It may also include a summary of any voluntary work or international experiences and particularly any experiences of independent learning that demonstrates developing personal autonomy. As indicated below, a profile put together for an interview should provide evidence of specific achievements and experiences, that are relevant to the post being applied for.

The new graduate portfolio

The student portfolio will have been geared towards fulfilling the requirements of the qualifying course. However, as a graduate it is time to reorganise the portfolio in favour of information that is important to employers, to supporting a career and to meeting HCPC standards. A current CV should be developed and include all employment, key activities and roles undertaken before entering professional education. Voluntary work and unpaid work experiences should be noted as well as other significant learning experiences and outcomes. Any special achievements as a student should be highlighted. Prospective employers will be interested in evidence of being able to initiate and complete activities that count as personal and professional development and show a commitment to ongoing learning. They will also be looking for people who can work in a team yet demonstrate professional autonomy and self-sufficiency.

After gaining the professional qualification, education and learning has to continue and should be recorded in the portfolio. However, this time there is choice as to what form the learning experiences take and when they occur. There may already be an action plan in place for the immediate and possibly longer term future to help consolidate previous learning at university. Most learning experiences in employment will have to be self-initiated (and funded as necessary) but there is a wide choice available, even if it just means reflecting on everyday practice and learning from critical incidents and other events. A portfolio should record activity and learning that has derived from reflections. A profile will be needed to showcase relevant information to support an application for a job and any interview that follows. If using an e-portfolio, it will be necessary to consider the best format for a profile that can be accessed at interview if necessary.

The practitioner portfolio

As a career progresses, different information becomes important. Putting a portfolio together might prompt questions such as the following:

- Have I gained any additional qualifications since gaining the professional award?
- Have I focused on developing any specialist expertise or advanced practice?
- Have I undertaken or contributed to any special project or served as a member of a project group?
- Have I served as a committee member for any service or professional body?
- Have I organised or coordinated any special event, for example a careers evening, open day, study day or conference?
- Have I had an internal promotion or taken on any additional responsibilities at work as a temporary measure?
- Have I given any talks on my field of practice or my service?
- Have I undertaken any teaching; have I supervised students' practice learning experiences or given lectures?
- Have I undertaken or contributed to any research?
- Have I prepared any leaflets or information for clients, service users or carers?
- Have I reviewed, audited or developed any part of my service?
- Have I introduced any new working methods or written protocols, policies or procedures?
- Have I written any articles, chapters or books for publication?
- Have I presented papers or posters at a conference?
- Have I engaged in any capacity with my professional body?

This is not an exhaustive list but hopefully it will prompt memories of experiences to note for future reference. It will help to gather the evidence of this activity, particularly where it is recent activity, in case it is ever needed for the CPD audit or to show any future employer. Whenever there is a significant new achievement to record, it is important to ensure that it is noted in the CV and not just as a reference within the portfolio.

Portfolios or profiles for interviews and promotion

As indicated above, a portfolio may have many uses, including the means of demonstrating how criteria for promotion or for a new job can be met. Some judgement will need to be made about the range and quantity of material necessary to support an interview for a new job. A detailed portfolio is usually unnecessary unless specifically requested. There is often little time to review a full portfolio at interview. A carefully constructed profile that targets specific evidence to meet the job criteria is preferable. Whilst much of the evidence within the portfolio might offer a composite picture of the applicant as a health professional, the key features of the portfolio should be selected according to the person specification that has been prepared by the employer for the job. As an applicant, it is critically important to demonstrate how the job criteria are met at both the application phase and again at interview. These will include reference to relevant qualifications, experience and personal attributes that match the essential and the desirable qualities listed on the person specification. The profile will be no substitute for the personal interview but should be able to complement it by showing the relevant assets that would be brought to the new employer.

Advancement within a service where pay banding is based on performance criteria will rely on appropriate evidence of the applicant having met the relevant criteria. Again, a profile may be used to demonstrate achievement of the criteria with evidence of the date when the criteria were shown to be met and confirmation from the person who made that judgement.

Portfolios for career development

The best way of keeping in touch with recommendations about portfolio development as a graduate is through the relevant professional body. Professional bodies also have a specific interest in the promotion, maintenance and development of professional standards so that the public can be assured of the competence of the membership. The professional bodies provide information to the members about the scope of practice of the profession and the relevant level of competence required in different situations. Professional bodies serve as a resource, providing guidance on CPD and relevant opportunities for post-qualifying education, training and for professional development activities. The scope of practice for most of the health and social care professions can be broken down into about six categories:

1. Direct contact work with service users and carers. This will also include supporting the education of students of the profession.
2. Advanced/specialist/consultant practice.
3. Service management.

4. Education.
5. Research.
6. Private practice and consultancy.

Contents of portfolios will inevitably reflect the current practice of the practitioner. The HCPC makes allowances for the variations in practice when assessing the professional development activities of individuals but still has to ensure that its CPD standards are met. Portfolios will need to include relevant development opportunities and outcomes that show benefits for service users so that an appropriate selection of activities can be extracted for a profile as and when required for audit.

Putting a portfolio together

Putting together a portfolio is not as daunting as it sounds. The first choice to be made is whether to keep a manual or e-portfolio, although some people may choose to keep both for convenience. Most people find it easier to start with putting together factual information such as information for the CV. The overall framework of the portfolio can be worked out later. The information required for a CV is personal information and contact details, then a historical record of education and work-related activity. Before putting together any information in a CV it is worth putting together a list of relevant activity. Collect details of the following, with relevant dates:

• Formal qualifications and awarding institution.
• Unpaid work experiences or placements.
• Voluntary work and other related activity.
• Employment record.
• Details of significant roles and responsibilities undertaken.
• Other professional activity, such as projects, publications, teaching experiences, research and events organised.

Some people choose to add very brief comment on the specific learning that has been derived from each experience. It is not uncommon to have a CV even as an undergraduate. It is certainly worth putting one together early in a career. However, some of those who choose to study later in life to become a health or social care practitioner may be putting a CV together for the first time much later in life. The CV of an undergraduate may focus on pre-employment information. The CV of a more experienced practitioner may be biased towards formal qualifications and employment records. It is appropriate to use discretion about what goes in a CV; however, any significant gaps in the CV may need to be explained. For example, time taken as maternity leave might be noted. At the end of the CV, a summary of key strengths and skills might be useful. The CV must be updated (and dated) regularly and redundant information deleted in order to keep the CV concise and well focused.

When applying for a job, applicants may or may not be encouraged to forward a CV with the application form. For parity in the recruitment process, most employers now ask for relevant information to be included in the organisation's application form. Employers rarely consider any additional information that is submitted unless it has been invited. The CV held within a portfolio will contain all necessary information. The appropriate information to include on the application form will need to be made with special reference to the expectations of the job.

Developing a portfolio

Portfolio learning encompasses retrospective and prospective approaches. The retrospective approach involves looking back at what has been done in order to identify and produce a record of past achievements, possibly with some commentary on the learning process and outcomes. The prospective approach involves looking forward and entering into a process of planning, creating and pursuing learning opportunities. Reflection and careful analysis will allow areas of further development to be identified so that plans can be made for new learning. In this way, portfolios offer individuals a unique opportunity to direct and monitor their own learning and development in support of their professional career. This systematic approach should link in specifically with any appraisal or performance review so that further career development is not lost in a system that otherwise focuses mainly on personal progress within an organisation.

There is no doubt that portfolio development is a necessary but time-consuming activity that requires individuals to be disciplined, systematic and thorough in their approach to identifying, recording and presenting relevant evidence of learning and development. Although it takes time to select, record and order the information, the portfolio becomes the central location for all information relevant to a career. Getting it right should save time and effort in the future. There may also be spin-offs as developing a portfolio can change the way in which learning is approached. It can help make individuals more analytical and critical of their own performance and more amenable to learning.

Taking a break from practice

Anyone considering taking a short break from practice should attempt to keep themselves up to date with practice in their profession by attending meetings, reading journals or undertaking other activity that can be managed in the circumstances. Maintaining a record of this activity in a portfolio will help support any preparations for returning to practice and for the HCPC audit, should it apply. In the United Kingdom, a deferral of 1 year can be sought from the HCPC in respect of the audit in certain circumstances. However, submission of the profile will normally be expected the following year. A career break of up to 2 years is not likely to impact on registration with the HCPC, but a longer break may mean that more specific criteria must be met before being granted registered status again. All relevant information is available on the HCPC website.

Returning to practice

Anyone wishing to return to practise in their profession after a considerable break in service should first acquaint themselves with the current expectations of the regulatory body for seeking and gaining registration. The professional body can also be a good source of information and may be able to provide details of any relevant 'return to practice' programmes that might be on offer. The HCPC would normally expect those returning to practise after a break of longer than 2 years to undertake a specified period of updating knowledge and skills. During that period a variety of activities may be undertaken, such as a combination of supervised practice, formal study and private study. During the period of updating, those seeking registration might be strongly advised to create (or update) a portfolio. Records of professional updating activity will need to be provided to the regulatory body, so the sooner these records are started the better. Once registered, the requirement to maintain a portfolio of professional development activities will apply. Any of the learning activities suggested in this book could be suitable and used for professional updating.

A checklist for your portfolio

This checklist is provided mainly for those who have chosen to keep a manual portfolio, although those using e-portfolios may still find the prompts helpful.
    Does the updated portfolio:

- contain an up-to-date CV?
- present records and evidence of CPD activities in a structured way?
- present information that is concise, comprehensive, clear, well ordered, indexed and cross-referenced as necessary?
- demonstrate reflection, analysis, critical awareness and self-evaluation?
- indicate learning outcomes from CPD activities?
- indicate how CPD activities have contributed to your professional development?
- describe how your CPD activities have impacted positively on service delivery, patient care and the needs of carers?
- offer personal development goals and plans for the future?

Professional development and career planning

A portfolio has some key functions that assist practitioners to manage professional development and show evidence of meeting HCPC registration and CPD requirements. It also serves as a reference point for a career. As a career progresses, it can be quite difficult to remember what activities or roles were undertaken at a particular time in professional development. The portfolio helps keep those records for reference as and when required. The portfolio also has a function to assist in your career planning. Not all personal aspirations will be shared with colleagues or line managers, but they can be noted in a portfolio and can be worked upon in private. Alternatively, some of these aspirations could be made public in, for example, a performance review situation when longer term personal and professional plans are discussed. Action plans that may incrementally support longer term career development plans can be set out. Therefore, it is important to plan and use the portfolio in ways best suited to personal needs and not just to maintain it for audit purposes. It is clear that there are direct links between keeping a portfolio and job-seeking, maintaining professional competence, meeting the requirements of the regulatory body, performance review, gaining promotion and career planning and development. It is thus important to view a portfolio as a positive record of personal strengths and achievements and as a proactive approach to keeping up to date and to developing skills and competence. Embedding future plans and progress reports within the portfolio should also create the evidence for the celebration of personal achievements.

Summary

This chapter has presented definitions of portfolios and profiles and considered their purpose with regard to recording and presenting information about continuing professional development (CPD) activity. Students of the health and social care professions are normally introduced to portfolios during their course leading to professional qualification with a view to their ongoing use in practice. The particular requirements of the UK regulatory body, the Health and Care Professions Council (HCPC), have been outlined with reference to audit of health and social care professionals' CPD. However, readers have been advised to consult the HCPC website for current and specific directions with regard to audit as these may change over time. Anyone taking a break from practice is advised to continue to maintain their CPD portfolio for future use. Various uses of portfolios have been considered including their use at interviews. Both manual and e-portfolios may be used to record activity that contributes to learning, professional development and preparation for promotion. Different ways of presenting material, for example in picture form, have also been discussed.

References

Brown RA (1992) *Portfolio Development and Profiling for Nurses*. Quay Publications, Lancaster.
Brown S & Knight P (1994) *Assessing Learners in Higher Education*. Kogan Page, London.
HPC (2010) *Continuing Professional Development and your Registration*. Health Professions Council, London.
Redman W (1994) *Portfolios for Development: A Guide for Trainers and Managers*. Kogan Page, London.

Chapter 4

The process of continuing professional development

This chapter addresses:

1. the professional journey as a learning career;
2. the process of continuing professional development (CPD);
3. coaching, mentorship, preceptorship and other networks as support mechanisms in professional practice.

Introduction

The professional career is a journey through which each professional travels at his or her own pace and in a direction that is largely self-determined. Much of the preparation for this journey takes place through a prescribed pre-registration qualifying programme in an educational establishment, but the real journey begins at the point of qualification. A professional career becomes a 'learning career', a lifelong learning process that includes the formal requirement of continuing professional development (CPD) to meet regulatory requirements. The CPD process is one that has to be steered by the professional, taking account of personal circumstances and the environmental context that offers the employment opportunities. Support mechanisms such as coaching and mentoring can provide help and guidance in support of career development.

The professional journey

The educational programme leading to a professional qualification is the first part of the professional journey that is guided by lecturers who ensure that the journey proceeds at an appropriate pace and in an appropriate way in order to achieve a satisfactory outcome for each learner. Even though each individual on that journey

Continuing Professional Development in Health and Social Care: Strategies for Lifelong Learning, Second Edition. Auldeen Alsop.
© 2013 John Wiley & Sons, Ltd. Published 2013 by John Wiley & Sons, Ltd.

will complete an approved course and meet the required professional standards, each member of the group will have different interests and gain different insights and benefits from the learning experiences to which they are exposed. Some may have had a previous career and are seeking a change or a chance to develop in a different direction. They will bring a range of expertise that will serve as a backdrop to their new learning. Others will be school leavers on the verge of their first career. So, even qualifiers in the same profession can have different profiles of skills and attributes at the start of their professional career. The main difference with the professional journey after qualification is that there is no guide. Each 'traveller' will have to be self-reliant and self-directed, planning and arranging different learning experiences for himself or herself according to personal needs, interests and professional aspirations. Some employers may provide support and direction for new graduates entering the workplace, for example in the form of preceptorship or through similar local arrangements. Other graduates who enter employment in less structured environments may find themselves having to set their own agenda from the start. Seeking out support mechanisms that can be tapped into at the start of a professional career will thus be a priority.

The first steps on the post-qualification career path are likely to include a period of consolidation of learning and of applying new found knowledge under the supervision of, or in consultation with, a more experienced practitioner. Such experiences can provide opportunities for ongoing learning in a less directed way and further develop competence and confidence for independent practice. Many health professionals, on graduating, will take up positions in health or social services and thus work within a well-established and structured environment that provides support, supervision and opportunities for further development. Other qualifying professionals may seek work in organisations where support mechanisms and opportunities for learning and advancement are less well developed. Tapping into some external support mechanisms may be crucial as an aid to development and to help minimise possible feelings of isolation especially when embarking on a new career. In non-statutory organisations, it should still be possible to identify someone who can guide performance through regular, structured learning conversations. If this is not possible, then seeking someone outside the organisation who could act as a mentor would be beneficial.

The newly qualified practitioner can expect to spend the next year or so consolidating practice and developing competence in the role of an autonomous, self-directed, reflective practitioner who is able to work creatively and take decisions based on independent professional judgement. This is not to say that all decisions must be taken independently of others. Part of the judgement will be to acknowledge personal limitations and to consult with other relevant people to obtain other views and opinions as necessary that will inform the decision-making process. Experts and peers from the same or other professions can input into the decision-making process, as can clients. Over time, experience might be gained in a number of different locations and the strengths and limitations of the different areas of practice will become apparent. The insights emerging from different work experiences are likely to inform personal decisions about the future direction of a career.

Envisioning a career

In the early stages of a professional career, it can be quite difficult to think of anything other than immediate goals of professional development to ensure that practice not only is consolidated but also continues to improve. Professional supervision and performance reviews or appraisals can offer opportunities to start thinking about longer term plans and development needs, although it is quite usual for views about career aspirations to emerge slowly over time. Often work experiences that do not offer personal satisfaction can help narrow the choices of a future career direction. Sometimes, it is easier to specify the areas of work that do not appeal – at least for the immediate future – than those that do appeal. Some practitioners come to love working with people of a particular age group, whilst others might select a preferred clinical specialty and take steps to gain expertise in the relevant area. Some practitioners want to see their practice skills develop so as to attain a high level of clinical expertise, whilst others see themselves heading towards management careers or a career in education or research. Practice, management, education and research tend to be the four key career areas open to a health or social care professional, although they are not mutually exclusive. A role drawing on two or more areas of expertise can be developed together and provide significant personal and professional satisfaction. However, the skills needed to perform well in specialist practice, service management, education or research must still be developed. Envisioning a career can help focus the mind on planning development opportunities that will help fulfil these personal goals.

Developing competence for a career

Career development requires individuals to build on their knowledge and skills and so enhance their level of competence from that attained during their initial professional education. Competence comprises a range of attributes that all need attention during the development process. Professional and technical knowledge and skills are all necessary for effective practice. Effective learning skills must also be in place so that professional development can occur. Learning skills and strategies are addressed in other chapters. However, it has to be noted that the motivation to learn, the preferred mode and pace of learning and the structure in which effective learning takes place will differ from individual to individual. Personal circumstances and personal aspirations may dictate the potential place and choice of development activities undertaken. All these will affect career development. Career development depends on the development of personal attributes as well as professional skills.

Personal development comes from a range of experiences through the roles we play in life, holidays that we take, books that we read, people that we meet and talk to and many other planned and unexpected personal experiences. We engage in lifelong learning even as we participate in everyday life, although we may not recognise that learning is taking place. Knowledge and personally constructed meaning from encounters are stored for later use. Personal learning includes developing confidence to operate effectively in a variety of circumstances, self-reliance, self-esteem and the skills of communication that assist with the building of rapport and working relationships with other people.

The process of CPD can take a number of forms dependent on whether the focus is on maintaining competence to practise for public protection in the current job, developing competence in a current or a new field of practice or developing oneself for career advancement and promotion. It is not that these are necessarily mutually exclusive, but maintaining competence will primarily focus on meeting regulatory standards in the short term. Developing competence or preparing for career advancement may entail taking a broad, longer term and personal view of CPD. Investing in oneself is both the purpose and reward of taking a longer term view of professional development within the scheme of a lifelong learning programme. Creating career options through a broader plan of CPD will benefit any individual working in a climate of constant change. As has already been said in Chapter 1, no job is for life, so creating ways of maximising employment opportunities in the workplace has to be advantageous.

The process of continuing professional development

The process of CPD is much the same as any other process designed to bring about change or improvement in a person's situation. The CPD process similarly involves:

- taking stock of current personal capability within the context of employment;
- assessing strengths, limitations, aspirations and needs;
- defining short and longer term goals within the context of a potential career;
- making realistic plans to undertake CPD activity in support of attaining desired outcomes and goals with due regard for personal circumstances and the needs of the current workplace;
- implementing the plan to achieve desired outcomes;
- evaluating the effectiveness of the process with reference to longer term goals;
- recording outcomes in terms of personal learning and benefits to service users;
- reviewing need and redefining the plan periodically.

Taking stock of one's own capability within the context of current employment would normally be facilitated by annual performance review with a line manager. Depending on the job role, intermittent case reviews may also take place as a mechanism of professional support and guidance within the workplace. These will be documented to form a formal record that accords with service expectations. Any such scheme provides the means by which performance is periodically reviewed and it can highlight any development need. An annual review of performance will examine previously set objectives that relate specifically to performance in the workplace and assess the extent to which these have been met. New objectives are likely to be set that indicate future development needs and goals for the forthcoming year. New objectives will be set in the context of the needs of the employing organisation and any changes that can be anticipated in service provision or work practices. For some newly qualified professionals, a six monthly review of performance and ongoing needs may be undertaken, possibly under preceptorship arrangements. Development needs are likely to relate to enhancing capacity to meet organisational goals, although they may also support general personal development needs. In addition to a formal performance review in the workplace, each individual should review wider personal expectations of future employment and associated development needs (for the shorter or longer term) in order to devise a more personalised development plan.

Assessing strengths, limitations, aspirations and needs can be done fairly readily. A practical way of doing this would be to use the four key headings to create and complete a table that addresses the four parameters. Strengths and limitations may be readily defined, especially within the context of any professional performance review that has taken place within the workplace. However, for the purpose of CPD planning personal aspirations should be explored so that a realistic development plan can be devised that helps to progress a wider career and not just the current job. Development needs can be specified and if necessary placed in some priority order.

Defining short-term objectives and longer term goals means creating some kind of vision of a preferred direction of a career. It need only be provisional as no one can anticipate the kinds of changes in the environmental context that might impact on personal aspirations and plans in the future. However, some professionals will be clear about their preferred direction of travel with regard to a career and set specific goals. These may indicate plans to study for a higher academic award or seek more specialised education and training so as to be able to focus on a more specialist or advanced area of practice within their profession. Others may focus on immediate expectations of career development within the existing workplace.

Making realistic plans will necessarily mean first taking stock of one's present personal and professional situation. Clearly, if CPD needs indicate action plans that relate specifically to the current work situation then appropriate plans will need to be identified. If career aspirations indicate preferences for specialisation or promotion, then plans may need to show step-by-step progression towards achieving longer term goals. In identifying plans it will be necessary to consider personal as well as professional circumstances. Is this the right time to be taking on, for example, further studies for a higher degree? Are there family or other carer commitments that may impact on studies? Could other shorter term plans fulfil some needs whilst personal issues are being addressed? Are the finances in place to support more extensive educational development?

Implementing the plan may bring its own challenges. Clearly, if CPD plans relate specifically to the context of employment then there should be some organisational support to enable the plans to be progressed. Support may be both financial and in terms of time allocated for the completion of agreed development activity. Plans that are intended to meet career development or other personal aspiration may not be as well supported from within the workplace. This may mean that the individual has to identify and commit personal resources in terms of finance and time outside of employment hours unless other sponsorship is forthcoming. There is still a personal responsibility to undertake the minimum developmental activity required for ongoing registration regardless of organisational support.

Evaluating the effectiveness of the learning process requires well-developed skills of critical reflection and evaluation. Every professional has a responsibility to maintain competence through continuous learning. CPD plans obtained from an appraisal, or set as a result of personal aspiration, will focus the mind on ways of gaining new knowledge and skills, but new learning has to be identified through a systematic process of reflection and review. Critically reflective skills should be used to examine carefully the extent to which development plans were fulfilled, the expected and unanticipated learning that emerged from engaging in the activity and the potential use of that new learning in practice.

Recording the learning that has taken place is imperative. Written evidence of successful completion of development plans needs to be maintained in readiness for the next appraisal in the workplace. Records should necessarily indicate personal reflections on the learning that has been achieved and ways in which that learning is being implemented in practice. For regulatory purposes, the record has to show that the new learning has benefited service provision and patient care management. Minimally, the learning derived from CPD will be recorded. However, unanticipated learning may also derive from experiences and the learning activities associated with those plans. These too should be recorded fully. Reflection on those experiences will highlight the learning generated from the new or unanticipated experiences. It is important to show how the new learning will contribute to professional growth.

Reviewing and revising the development plan will necessarily take account of all anticipated and unanticipated learning from the previous review period. It will also take account of the present context of employment and your place within it. Over the course of a year (a normal period between appraisals), the wider political, environmental, social and technological contexts may have changed considerably and these may have such a significant impact on employment prospects and career aspirations that completely new plans for professional development may have to be made. Personal circumstances may also have changed, either freeing you up to pursue new avenues of a career or placing new constraints on you whereby plans may have to be completely revised.

Preceptorship

In the United Kingdom, some professions such as nursing and occupational therapy have adopted the process of preceptorship to facilitate the early stages of professional development of new graduates within the relevant profession (Morley, 2006, 2007, 2009). Morley (2006) describes a preceptor as a role model or resource person within the clinical setting; someone who is assigned to support a new graduate during the early days of his or her first post within the health service. The aim is to facilitate the transition of the new graduates into employment as they deal with the stress and uncertainties of their new role. Preceptors can also assist with the development of new skills and knowledge and help consolidate professional identity. The challenges faced by new graduates of the health professions have also been recognised, although less formally, in countries such as Canada and Australia where recommendations have been put forward for appropriate support mechanisms to be put in place.

For newly qualified occupational therapists joining the NHS, the preceptorship programme lasts for about a year with specific targets set for the first 6 months. Following a review of progress, a revised list of objectives is set for the second 6 months. These targets align with expectations of the NHS Knowledge and Skills Framework (DH, 2004) so that new graduates working within the NHS are facilitated to work towards achieving nationally recognised goals. The standards set for the preceptorship programme for occupational therapists are given as follows:

- Working with clients or groups.
- Working with colleagues and other agencies.
- Written communication.
- Using local clinical policies relating to working practice.

Additionally, there is a set of professional behaviours to be demonstrated (Morley, 2009). The preceptorship cycle (Morley, 2007) follows the experiential learning cycle of Kolb (1984) and can be used by the preceptor and new graduate to assess knowledge and skills, and then to plan, implement and reflect on activity to improve performance. The cycle for professional growth (Morley, 2007) is a similar framework for CPD.

Coaching and mentorship

The terms coaching and mentoring have sometimes been used interchangeably but Parsloe (1995) distinguished between the two roles. He noted the origins of the two words as a useful starting point. Coaching, he suggested, is derived from university slang for private tutoring or instruction in sport, whereas mentoring has its origins in advising and counselling. For centuries, according to Darwin (2000) mentoring has been used as a medium for handing down knowledge and supporting talent. Therefore, coaching is directly concerned with the immediate improvement of performance and the development of skills, whereas mentoring is concerned with the longer term acquisition and application of skills in a developing career. Both a coach and mentor can facilitate learning but the opportunities for, and the range and direction of, learning might be different. Both can assist with determining a vision for a future career and both can help develop the skills needed to achieve ambitions and goals. However, a coach could be a colleague or line manager whereas a mentor should normally be someone who is distanced from direct line management arrangements. Coaching partnerships normally cease if one of the partners leaves the service whereas mentoring arrangements can continue to exist even when the employment situation of either person changes.

Coaching is said to be a process in which, through discussion and guided activity, a manager helps a member of staff to solve a problem, carry out or complete a task better (Kalinauckas, 1995). This involves the learner and coach exploring an opportunity or a problem together and then the coach enables the learner to develop new knowledge, skills and competencies through working on the problem (Pedlar et al., 1997). Coaching tends to use the process of modelling, exposing the learner to the way in which an expert thinks, reasons and makes decisions. Reflection on the process facilitates learning and the integration of new knowledge and skills into subsequent practice. According to Kalinauckas, the focus of coaching is on practical improvement of performance and on the development of specific skills. He goes on to describe 'achievement coaching' as a continuous and participative process whereby the coach provides both the opportunity and encouragement for the learner to address his or her needs effectively in the context of personal and organisational objectives. A coach might:

- help clarify learning goals and set targets;
- talk through the task;
- demonstrate the competence required;
- demonstrate use of technology or particular skills;
- encourage reflection on the process;
- give feedback on performance;
- help explore and use mistakes constructively;
- encourage further self-monitoring;
- respond to any doubts expressed by the learner.

Kalinauckas (1995) asserted that coaching is about bringing out the best in people through an exploration of their personal vision, values and beliefs and linking these to the vision, values and beliefs of the organisation. Therefore, everyone should gain from the relationship and the learning process. However, it tends to be a narrower and more focused relationship than that with a mentor.

Various definitions of 'mentor' exist. Wright and Sugarman (2009, p. 184) define a mentor as 'an influential role model who also serves directly as an informal guide or adviser in relation to the protégé's occupational and/or personal values, goals, [and] behaviours'. Megginson and Clutterbuck (1995) initially suggested that the mentorship relationship was about counselling and sharing knowledge with the protégé with a view to improving performance and supporting career development. However, they later defined mentoring as 'the seized opportunity to develop personal insight through uninterrupted and purposeful reflective activity' (Clutterbuck & Megginson, 1999, p. 8). This is an interesting definition as it moves the relationship from an advisory to a facilitatory one by initially encouraging the protégé to reflect on his or her performance. The relationship thus becomes 'learner-driven' (Megginson & Whitaker 2007, p. 123). The choice of mentor becomes critical as the mentee must be able to develop a positive and productive working relationship with the mentor in order to gain from the mentoring process. Whereas once a mentor might have been viewed as a trusted counsellor, teacher or guide, nowadays a mentor is more likely to use adult learning principles with the mentee to enable learning through a reflective process that prompts self-evaluation of performance and critical analysis of potential ways forward.

A mentor is concerned with the development of the person throughout a career or lifetime using active listening and questioning techniques and prompting reflection to help develop and enlarge a person's awareness both of self and of the wider world. According to Darwin (2000), the development of knowledge has to be viewed as an active process in which curiosity is encouraged and where learning becomes a dynamic, reciprocal and participatory process. The mentor thus stimulates professional development. He or she might help the protégé to:

- develop a personal vision of a future career;
- assess needs and establish a personal and professional development plan;
- recognise personal assets as well as gaps in experience;
- test out, in confidence, a range of ideas and working methods prior to making a decision about a way forward;
- explore and develop ideas;
- reflect on past performance and identify strengths and limitations;
- critically examine any given guidance and constructive feedback;
- question and challenge assumptions;
- develop self-confidence and self-reliance;
- build a sense of personal identity.

The mentoring relationship thus provides emotional support as well as helps to develop knowledge and skills. Darwin (2000, p. 204) sees the mentor as 'a transitional figure who guides and nurtures the protégé into the adult world through a series of phases, from dependence to independence'. Mentorship is nevertheless a professional relationship that can promote development and growth throughout a career. The choice of mentor is thus critical and the parameters of the relationship must be clear and respected by both parties. In selecting a mentor, the protégé must seek someone who they respect and can work with. It is important that the protégé can seek guidance but can ultimately retain control of decisions with regard to their career. Any relationship that does not work out should be terminated. Roth and Esdaile (2003) suggested the use of multiple mentors, rather than a single mentoring relationship. In this way, support is provided by a number of different people who all assist in the development of the protégé. Each may have different strengths and different perspectives, experiences and expertise that may aid professional development, but with multiple mentoring the focus is more likely to be on learning than on interpersonal support. The protégé would have to manage the various support mechanisms and ensure that mentorship, however provided, ultimately supports the achievement of goals and enables career development.

Networks

Roth and Esdaile (2003) also explore the concept of networking as a means of forming and utilising relationships with others for the purpose of learning. Groups of people who work in the same clinical specialty may meet from time to time to engage in learning activity, for example to explore a published article, to share research, to discuss unusual clinical cases or in other ways further their understanding of specialist practice. Undertaking learning activity with the multi-disciplinary team or during uni-professional specialist meetings or conferences also constitutes net-working. Informal conversations with others working in a similar specialist area can be as useful as more formal learning sessions. Reflection on the conversations will highlight the learning that has transpired and that should be documented. Technology can support communication such as teleconferencing to maximise opportunities for those working at a distance to participate in informal conversations as well as more formal learning events without the need to travel. Connecting with people nation-ally and internationally who share common interests and use each other as sounding boards for problem-solving or for developing ideas that can enhance practice can be helpful for both career and service development. Some professional bodies facilitate the formation and support of specialist interest groups not only to bring like-minded people together for sharing their expertise but also to promote research that may benefit service users and raise the profile of the profession through making a new contribution to service delivery. Other networks include peer support networks. For example, new graduates who disperse to different employment positions on comple-tion of the qualifying programme may remain in contact for mutual support. Other peer support mechanisms may develop with individuals from different professions working at the same employment level in the same organisation. These can also serve as professional networks of people who are likely to understand issues emerging from the work environment and can reflect on the impact of the issues arising.

Individual performance review

Individual performance review (IPR), sometimes known as personal appraisal, is a quality assurance mechanism that serves to improve organisational effectiveness by reflecting on past performance and developing specific plans for future performance of individual employees. The system varies from organisation to organisation but the aims are very much the same. Normally, the local human resources department sets out the requirements of the performance review system and line managers put the system into operation. Each member of staff will have a review, normally annually, with their designated manager using the framework of performance review. The strengths and limitations of each employee and their development plans are identified so that staff competence and expertise can be developed and used to best advantage in and for the organisation.

Each employee is required to participate in the local scheme. It should be viewed as a positive process that genuinely sets out to identify the individual's strengths, limitations and development needs within a framework that is supportive of the individual. It should aid personal career development as well as focus on ensuring that appropriate skills and expertise are available to the organisation to serve the needs of its clients. Normally the line manager would set a date with the individual employee for the performance review, allowing sufficient time for the employee to reflect on progress and performance since joining the organisation, or since the last review, as appropriate. There is usually a form to be completed initially by the employee and then by the manager. The information on the form provides the focus for discussion around performance. Generally, the process allows for:

- a review of recent performance, taking account of any previously identified objectives;
- an acknowledgement of good performance and evaluation of its relevance to service delivery;
- a discussion around any areas of concern or difficulties encountered in achieving previously set objectives;
- a discussion around new skills that require development or skills that require further development to meet service needs;
- a discussion around longer term career plans and goals and potential ways in which these may be addressed within the organisation;
- the identification of new objectives for the forthcoming year and a discussion around plans, actions or activities that might assist with meeting the objectives.

The meeting held to review your performance should be located in a quiet environment free from distractions or interruptions from other members of staff or phone calls. It should be conducted in private so that you can have a confidential discussion about your work, and the meeting should be scheduled for sufficient time so as not to rush the discussion. Normally, an hour and a half or longer would be allocated for the meeting. The process should allow for a two-way constructive exchange of information and ideas. Ideally, you should be given the chance first to review your own performance. This gives you the opportunity to acknowledge your strengths and achievements and to explore significant factors that have facilitated your performance and satisfactory achievement of goals. It is important to reflect on the positive aspects of your performance first and to have those confirmed by your line manager. An exploration of any elements of practice that have been less successful should be tackled next. An honest critique of performance, first from you and then from your manager, should lead to an open discussion about any factors that have inhibited performance and resulted in a less successful outcome than expected. There may be valid reasons for the outcome, which should be noted.

Overall, IPR should be an enabling process that provides focused support to promote your professional development so that you are an asset to the organisation for which you work. Future plans and goals should be negotiated jointly. An action plan should set out objectives for the forthcoming year and the future direction that any development activity should take. Development activity should ensure that you remain safe and competent to practise in your position of employment and can meet requirements for re-registration with the regulatory body. Development plans could involve deployment in a different department or area of practice to broaden your experience, taking on additional responsibilities, attending a staff development programme or other ways to help you to progress in your career. If you are working as a registered practitioner in your organisation then opportunities for CPD to meet ongoing registration requirements may come up in discussion. CPD activity that supports service provision may be agreed and supported with study leave and, exceptionally, with financial support. However, there is no obligation on the organisation to provide such support. CPD to meet the requirements of the regulatory body is entirely the responsibility of the professional.

Summary

This chapter has considered the track of a professional career from the structured educational qualifying programme to the choices that present to individuals with regard to their future career. It is acknowledged that professionals have different backgrounds and personal profiles when first entering the profession and will have different career goals. Individual practitioners may choose to remain in practice providing health or social care services to the general public. However, some may also look to achieve career satisfaction in management, education or research. The process of continuing professional development (CPD) is explored. Individuals are encouraged to take stock of their situation and take responsibility for their own professional development with their career goals in mind. Performance review mechanisms may help clarify an individual's strengths and limitations in practice and any professional development needs. Although some CPD has to be completed to meet regulatory requirements and some may need to be completed as required by the employing organisation, taking personal control of CPD will also help professionals attain personal career goals. There are several other mechanisms that might provide support and guidance to individuals as they pursue their career. These include coaching, mentorship, preceptorship and other professional networks.

References

Clutterbuck D & Meginson D (1999) *Mentoring Executives and Directors*. Butterworth-Heinemann, Oxford.

Darwin A (2000) Critical reflections on mentoring in work settings. *Adult Education Quarterly*, **50** (3), 197–211.

DH (2004) *The NHS Knowledge and Skills Framework (NHS KSF) and the Development Review Process, Final Version*. Department of Health, London.

Kalinauckas P (1995) Coaching for CPD. In: *Continuing Professional Development – Perspectives on CPD in Practice* (ed. S Clyne), pp. 133. Kogan Page, London.

Kolb D (1984) *Experiential Learning: Experience as a Source of Learning and Development*. Prentice Hall, Englewood Cliffs, NJ.

Megginson D & Clutterbuck D (1995) *Mentoring in Action*. Kogan Page, London.

Megginson D & Whitaker V (2007) *Continuing Professional Development*, 2nd edn. Chartered Institute of Personnel and Development, London.

Morley M (2006) Moving from student to new practitioner: the transitional experience. *British Journal of Occupational Therapy*, **69** (5), 231–233.

Morley M (2007) Building reflective practice through preceptorship: the cycles of professional growth. *British Journal of Occupational Therapy*, **70** (1), 40–42.

Morley M (2009) *The Preceptorship Handbook for Occupational Therapists*, 2nd edn. College of Occupational Therapists, London.

Parsloe E (1995) *Coaching, Mentoring and Assessing: A Practical Guide to Developing Competence*. Kogan Page, London.

Pedlar M, Burgoyne J & Boydell T (1997) *The Learning Company: A strategy for Sustainable Development*, 2nd edn. McGraw-Hill, London.

Roth L & Esdaile S A (2003) Role models and mentors: informal and formal ways to learn from exemplary practice. In: *Becoming an Advanced Healthcare Practitioner* (eds G Brown, SA Esdaile & SE Ryan), pp. 239–259. Butterworth-Heinemann, Oxford.

Wright R & Sugarman L (2009) *Occupational Therapy and Life Course Development: A Workbook for Professional Practice*. John Wiley & Sons, Chichester.

Chapter 5

Learning to learn

This chapter addresses:

1. early learning and the development of the autonomous learner and autonomous practitioner;
2. evaluation of learning needs and developing competence to learn;
3. reflection as an aid to learning.

Introduction

Career development requires individuals to build on their knowledge and skills to develop their level of competence to practise, not just for ongoing registration but also for personal career satisfaction. As has been discussed, competence embraces many professional and technical skills and personal qualities necessary for effective practice. It also has to include skills for effective learning so that professional development can continue to take place. Therefore, competence to learn should be seen as integral to competence to practise.

Learning takes many forms over the course of a lifetime, from pre-school experiences, through formal education and into adulthood. Some initial learning is innate, and then as we grow, we learn through mimicking and through modelling our behaviour on that of others. We learn through play and through experimentation in different situations both alone and with others. Our parents and teachers guide and encourage us, praising us when things go well, redirecting us when we stray, so shaping our behaviour and what we come to know about the world. Play provides the building blocks for later life and enables us to seek explanations of the world and our place within it. Young people develop capacities through learning with and from others, from practising and refining skills and by using minds and bodies to enable survival. All forms of learning combine to help us decide on and manage future life roles.

Learning and other personal development activities have much to contribute to professional development. Personal development comes from a range of experiences

Continuing Professional Development in Health and Social Care: Strategies for Lifelong Learning,
Second Edition. Auldeen Alsop.
© 2013 John Wiley & Sons, Ltd. Published 2013 by John Wiley & Sons, Ltd.

through the roles we play in life, holidays that we take, books that we read, leisure activities that we engage with, the people we meet and talk to and many other planned and unexpected personal experiences. We participate in lifelong learning as we participate in everyday life even though we may not even recognise that learning is taking place. Personal learning includes developing confidence, self-esteem and the skills of communication that assist with the building of rapport and working relationships with other people. Knowledge and personally constructed meaning from encounters are stored for later use. So much of our future depends on learning that learning might be perceived as an occupation in its own right, that is, meaningful activity that takes up our time and energy, and brings its own rewards.

Griffin and Brownhill (2001) have claimed that lifelong learning means not only that individuals continue to learn over the whole of their lives but also that every aspect of their lives presents opportunities for learning. Formal and informal learning throughout early and teenage years helps shape us and helps to guide us towards a trade or profession that captures our interest, one that we believe can potentially make best use of our attributes and talents in adult life. Formal, often structured education and training lead to initial qualifications. Thereafter, the responsibility for further learning in order to maintain or enhance competence for work is ours alone. The mode and pace of learning and the structure in which learning takes place are likely to differ for each individual; nevertheless, learning will be ongoing. It is up to the individual how learning experiences are captured and used, and the extent to which learning progresses. This is likely to depend on each individual's capacity and motivation to learn, level of commitment to self-development and the degree to which skills and strategies for learning are in place. However, for health and social care professionals, the commitment to ongoing learning in order to remain competent and to develop competence and expertise is not an option but a legal and professional responsibility, so learning in some form must continue. The first stage is to develop helpful learning strategies as a student.

The student learner

Primarily, a course leading to a qualification in one of the health or social care professions will meet specific, recognised standards set down by the regulatory and professional bodies and meet the criteria for a graduate academic award. Students are commonly introduced to a range of learning strategies that include both academic and practice learning to ensure that they develop appropriate knowledge, skills and attitudes for professional practice. Underpinning the philosophy of learning is the need to develop autonomous learners who can take control of their own learning needs and instigate ways of developing themselves professionally during and after initial professional education. Authors such as Brookfield (1986) and Boud (1988) have suggested strategies for developing autonomous learners as preparation for autonomy in practice. Autonomous learners are considered to be those who are able to self-assess learning needs, able to select from a range of learning strategies and options to fulfil needs and, through self-directed learning processes, able to fulfil those needs.

Autonomous learners are thus considered to be those who are:

- competent to learn and able to operate with confidence in new and complex situations;
- intrinsically motivated to learn;
- able to determine learning needs and in control of decisions to address them;
- able to select ways of addressing needs from a range of known learning strategies;
- self-aware and able to implement learning strategies to attain goals;
- able to critically reflect on learning experiences to determine personal strengths, newly acquired knowledge and skill and further learning needs;
- able to self-regulate and adapt their approach to learning according to circumstances;
- able to use various technological resources to facilitate independent learning;
- able to enjoy learning and gain pleasure from the learning experience itself.

McNair (1996) argues that autonomous learners are efficient learners as they have a strong sense of self, understand why they are learning and have the confidence and capability to achieve the result. They are perceived as individuals with personal expectations and life plans (Watson, 1992) and thus with commitment to learning. Health and social care graduates should expect to leave university with the above capabilities as these are integral skills for practice development and for ongoing learning.

Identifying learning needs

Self-evaluation of development needs is an essential feature of a process that underpins professional development. The newly qualified practitioner who is able to assess and take steps to meet learning needs may advance readily through different stages of development within their career. The Skill Acquisition Model of Dreyfus and Dreyfus (1986) is sometimes used to illustrate progression in the development of tacit knowledge and the ability to apply it in practice (Eraut, 2005). Dowie and Elstein (1988, p. 95) have presented the key features of the five stages of Dreyfus and Dreyfus' model, which have been summarised in Table 5.1. In this model, learners may progress through the stages of development, namely novice, advanced beginner, competent, proficient and expert. Each stage has a particular set of attributes associated with capability that aligns with professional development leading ultimately to the ability to operate intuitively as an expert in practice.

The novice-to-expert continuum helps us to understand where we are in our own professional development and to define our needs and expectations regarding ongoing learning. It is possible to be both a novice and expert at the same time in different areas of practice, depending on how far expertise has been developed in each area. On qualification, a practitioner's skills may vary with some being below par even though overall the regulatory body's standards relating to their profession have been

Table 5.1   Stages of professional development.

Stage of development	Characteristics of the individual
Expert	A practitioner who no longer relies on rules: • has clear vision based on reflective experience; • has an intuitive grasp of situations; • makes decisions intuitively.
Proficient	A practitioner who has a sense of direction and vision: • sees situations holistically, not as components; • discriminates between important and less important information; • perceives situations intuitively; • makes strategic decisions analytically; • modifies action as situation changes.
Competent	A practitioner who can just cope in practice: • combines perception and action; • thinks analytically about whole situation; • plans deliberately and consciously; • tends to follow some procedures routinely.
Advanced beginner	A practitioner with some limited experience: • is still learning to distinguish between sets of information; • applies other people's rules to practice.
Novice	Someone with little or no experience: • thinks analytically about components of practice; • refers to guiding principles; • follows other people's rules.

met. On progression, levels of competence may develop significantly in selected areas of practice, through a state of proficiency to a level of expertise whereby the individual will be regarded as a specialist. However, for an individual, some skills may become highly developed, others may remain underdeveloped and some may fade. Competence, proficiency and expertise become intertwined as the practitioner claims a breadth of knowledge and skills but at different levels of understanding for each aspect of his or her work. Sometimes practitioners may opt to develop skills as a generalist and gain proficiency in a broad range of skill areas. This may arise as a result of opportunity (or lack of opportunity) for professional development in employment or because the individual has made an informed decision to develop him or herself in this way. Learning strategies can be put into place to suit the generalist or specialist, depending on the need or desire for breadth or depth of skill development. Knowing how to learn facilitates the planning of professional development in such a way that it reflects personal needs and enhances career prospects.

Learning as a dimension of competence

The newly qualified practitioner leaves university having been socialised into his or her chosen profession, having developed adequate professional knowledge and skills for competent performance, having an understanding of professional principles and ways in which they are applied in practice, having developed reasoning skills for making competent professional judgements and having developed the skills for ongoing professional development. The responsibility for lifelong learning is thus reinforced as a conscious commitment to ongoing learning that has to be taken seriously. Competence to learn is thus essential not only for developing competence to practise but also for engaging successfully in continuing professional development (CPD). Competence in learning is about having a positive attitude to education, taking initiatives to learn, being open to new methods of practice, and about seizing learning opportunities and working with new ideas and concepts to improve professional performance. It is about developing the skills to question and reflect on practice, to evaluate one's own performance and to accept and respond to constructive feedback. Knowing how to use learning resources, taking opportunities to practise and refine skills and knowing when and where to seek help and guidance are all features of effective learning.

The skills to locate and use different learning resources, including technological resources, will have been developed during initial professional education and can be drawn on again for CPD purposes. The time for exploring learning resources in practice has to be built into any strategy for professional development as the resources in practice may not be as readily available or accessible as those in education establishments. If skills in using learning resources need to be updated, the first port of call might be a library or learning centre. Technology, in particular, is changing at such a pace that it is difficult to keep up to date with all resources that can support learning. Competence in using technological resources efficiently and effectively will help in the location and management of learning materials and may save hours of work in the longer term. The use of social media as a means of tapping into the thoughts and perceptions of colleagues both nationally and internationally could also be developed to support learning. Practitioners who are returning to work after a considerable period of absence may need to gain an understanding of how new forms of communication can assist learning and CPD. The more that novice practitioners understand about the function of learning in relation to developing competence and confidence for practice, the sooner will they have the personal attributes to operate as autonomous practitioners.

The autonomous practitioner

During professional education, students are introduced to the concept of learner autonomy and to learning techniques that encourage them to become autonomous learners in readiness for autonomy in practice. The need to develop and operate as an autonomous practitioner has been advocated for quite some time. In 1996, McNair indicated that working careers were becoming more complex and unpredictable and that external support for individuals to be able to develop in the workplace was becoming less reliable. Therefore, professionals needed to learn quickly to work independently and make autonomous decisions for survival in these environments.

The confidence and expertise to think, make decisions and act autonomously (Creek, 2007) has to be built up during the early stages of a professional career, starting at the level of the student practitioner. Professional qualifying education should enable students to develop an awareness of multiple perspectives and to use different learning and decision-making strategies in practice. Both students and newly qualified practitioners should be afforded the opportunity to try out new ideas in practice and to use different strategies to problem solve in order to build up confidence, competence and professional expertise with due regard for patient safety and autonomy. There is a need for practitioners to work towards being self-reliant so that they can find ways independently of coping with all manner of challenges in practice. The key to their learning, as always, is to ensure that they have opportunity for reflection on experiences soon after the event in order to assess the relative merits of their chosen strategy, any learning that has occurred in the process and any future development needs. A line manager, mentor or critical friend might assist in this process.

Learning from experience

Eraut (2002) suggested that, after we finish with formal education, most of what we learn is likely to stem from experience. This informal learning from experience tends to be a much less conscious process than formal education in the classroom. Learning experiences are accumulated over time and aggregated to provide the overall capacity to deal with increasingly more complex practice situations. However, the learning from these experiences will be significantly enhanced by undertaking some critical and analytical reflection on what has occurred. This is particularly so where unique and uncertain situations have been encountered and where personal decision-making has been significantly put to the test (Megginson & Whitaker, 2007). A systematic reflective review can help reassure autonomous decision-making capacity as well as help diagnose personal decision-making problems that still need to be addressed.

Reflection

Brookfield (1986) argued that merely selecting an appropriate learning strategy was insufficient to achieve the desired learning. The most complete form of self-directed learning occurs 'when process and reflection are married in the adult's pursuit of meaning' (Brookfield, 1986, p. 58). Critical reflection and exploration of different perspectives and meanings are thus crucial to the learning process. These can lead to some reinterpretation of the personal and social world. Critical reflection can be undertaken alone, but there may be more benefit from participating in a reflective discussion with another person. Learning from different experiences where choice has been exercised can underpin the development of professional artistry (Andresen & Fredericks, 2001), that is, the capacity to operate creatively and flexibly, as necessary, within a practice tradition but according to individual circumstances. Experts intuitively use artistry in its many forms, including improvisation, in order to meet the needs of clients when more traditional practice strategies may be inappropriate or liable to fail.

Much of the theory related to adult learning stresses the value of using reflection to discover the meaning of new experiences and the learning that has been derived from them. New learning depends on making new discoveries, seeing new connections and relationships and thus gaining new insights and knowledge from particular situations. Many theorists have offered models of reflection. All in some way entail creating a story of an experience and then asking critical questions about the event and its consequences. Firstly, the following definition of reflection is helpful with regard to its link to learning:

> Reflection in the context of learning is a generic term for those intellectual and affective activities in which individuals engage to explore their experiences in order to lead to new understandings and appreciation (Boud et al., 1985, p. 19).

Although Schön (1983) noted that professionals both reflect-in-action and reflect-on-action, most learning probably derives from reflection-on-action.

Reflection can be used in various ways after different learning experiences. For learning events that are intentional in that they are pre-planned and often pursued through organised forms of learning, reflection is part of the systematic process of the cycle of learning. After the event, it is worth spending some time thinking back over the activities to identify new knowledge, skills and perspectives that have emerged and that will make a difference to future practice. Conversations with others about the learning experience are likely to identify even more perspectives that can also contribute to learning.

A structured series of questions that guide reflection on an action can help focus the learning strategy (Johns, 2002). The questions are concerned with both events and emotions in order to critically examine what happened and what might be learnt from the experience. Sometimes negative emotions can interfere with the process, so Johns suggests a focus on positive factors. Figure 5.1 reflects a modified version of Johns' model. This structured approach may be useful for recording incidents that

---

Reflect on experiences by addressing the following:
- Recount the experience as a story (verbally or in writing)
- Identify the issues that seem significant in some way
- How was I feeling at the time and what made me feel that way?
- What was I trying to achieve?
- Did I respond effectively and in line with my values?
- What were the consequences of my actions on others and for me?
- How were others feeling, and what made them feel that way?
- What factors influenced how I was feeling?
- How does this situation connect with any previous experiences?
- How might I respond more effectively another time?
- How do I now feel about the experience?
- Do I need to take any further action to supplement my learning from this experience?

Figure 5.1   A model for structured reflection (adapted from Johns 2002)

Consider:
- What went well – and why?
- What did not go so well – and why?
- What did other people say about the incident?
- So what have I learnt?
- What would I do differently next time?

Figure 5.2   A quick model of reflection

might be put forward as learning scenarios within a profile prepared for a regulatory body audit of CPD.

For everyday practice, a shortened version might aid reflection and learning from experiences in practice. The questions to be asked about an incident are shown in Figure 5.2. The questions in Figure 5.2 can be reflected upon quite quickly. They may still offer new insights into experiences from which learning might occur. Both versions are suitable for supervisors to use with students or line managers to use with newly qualified practitioners. The adapted version from Johns (Figure 5.1) encourages a deeper and broader understanding of significant events and lends itself to a written version that can later be discussed in some depth with a supervisor, line manager or mentor. The model in Figure 5.2 could be used by a student or practitioner either independently or to form the basis of a quick debrief following an event or incident in practice.

Learning can also take place in less structured and often unanticipated ways. These experiences occur often by chance and sometimes catch us unaware. Time to reflect on these unexpected but novel experiences that often occur in everyday life can reveal new insights that contribute to experiential learning. Connections can often be made between two or more unrelated experiences. Again, attention should be paid to the affective element of the experience, as this is where very personal learning can occur. In a similar way to other theorists, Boud et al. (1993) considered that reflection comprised a number of processes whereby learners recapture, notice and re-evaluate their experience, work with the experience and turn it into learning. Revisiting the experience in our mind, taking note of the key features of the event, exploring for ourselves what happened and what the consequences are, and establishing how this adds to, or changes, what we already know, is the essence of reflection. Insights gained from one experience might then be drawn on in future situations. The focus here is reflection on unplanned learning experiences that contribute to personal and professional development. Both planned and unplanned learning experiences have their place on the CPD agenda.

Reflective practice as a health or social care practitioner has also to be mastered for learning purposes to improve the service offered to clients and service users. Boud (1989) maintained that one of the defining characteristics of a professional's work was the need and ability to monitor personal performance. This could be done through a process of self-evaluation that involved critical assessment of personal performance, the monitoring of progress and the determination of meaningful learning goals (Boud, 1992). Self-evaluation is thus a process that underpins professional development. However, self-evaluation could not be completed without reflection. Reflection on performance assists practitioners to recapture the experiences they have had, to think about them, ponder over and evaluate them in a systematic way so that strengths, limitations and aspects of performance that need improvement can be identified (Boud et al., 1996). As Cross et al. (2006) noted, using reflection is an active process that leads to enhanced knowledge and understanding of performance. It enables the learner to acquire new perspectives on practice and to become more self-aware as a self-directed learner. The new learning that derives from the process should confirm aspects of professional practice that are improving as well as highlight those that require further development.

Learning as an investment

Each one of us will have personal aspirations and goals for the future even though they may not all relate to professional or career development. These affect our commitment to learning and skill development. For example, some people may consider taking a break from professional practice to return to full-time study, to travel or to become a full-time parent or carer. Some may be content to balance a social life with work, possibly working part time, and just keep sufficiently abreast of the changes that affect practice to maintain a professional role. Others will have a commitment to develop professionally, to update professional knowledge and to develop expertise and skills in order to advance in a career. Whatever the plan, an element of learning is likely to be involved.

Uncertainty about employment could also mean that individuals need to consider moving between jobs during their working life. Learning to manage these transitions successfully is also important. Health and social care practitioners are not immune to the challenges and changes in the political and economic climate and the disruption to employment opportunities. Health and social care is subject to frequent reorganisation. Some posts can be lost or transformed into new posts requiring different skills. Redeployment of professionals into different, and perhaps more challenging, positions is not unknown. The geographical terrain in some places could mean that some professionals find themselves working single-handed in fairly isolated situations. More than ever before, in order to cope with these challenges, individuals need to be able to work autonomously and draw on their enterprise skills, their willingness to be flexible and their ability to be creative in both existing and new places of work.

Developing knowledge and skills should not just be considered for immediate gain but as an investment for the future. Whatever the goal, it is perceived that adults like to be in control of their learning so that they can choose the pace and means of addressing their learning needs. All previous experience will influence and shape attitudes to any new learning challenge (Cross et al., 2006). Attitudes to learning and personal motivation to learn will thus influence the way in which CPD expectations are met. Conversations about personal and professional development with a mentor, or a discussion about current and future practice with a line manager during supervision or individual performance review could highlight gaps in knowledge or skill and help with focusing the choice of learning and CPD initiatives.

Summary

This chapter considers learning as an occupation in which we engage throughout life. Initial learning is innate, prompted by the need to survive. Youngsters learn through play as curiosity encourages them to explore the environment under the guidance of parents. Personal development comes from a range of life experiences including formal and informal learning. In the academic environment, students of the professions are guided towards developing skills for autonomous learning in order to prepare them for working as an autonomous practitioner. Learning includes mastering the location and use of resources, including technological resources to support learning and professional development. Learning strategies include experiential learning and taking the time to reflect on learning activities. The development of professional competence comes in different phases, from novice to expert. Competence to learn is integral to competence to practise and must continue to feature highly throughout professional life. Given the frequency of changes in the external environment, learning to work autonomously, to be flexible and manage transitions is seen as an investment for future employment.

References

Andresen L & Fredericks I (2001) Finding the fifth player: artistry in professional practice. In: *Professional Practice in Health, Education and the Creative Arts* (eds J Higgs & A Titchen), pp. 72–89. Blackwell Science, Oxford.

Boud D (ed.) (1988) Moving towards autonomy. In: *Developing Student Autonomy in Learning*, 2nd edn, pp. 17–39. Kogan Page, London.

Boud D (1989) The role of self-assessment in student grading. *Assessment and Evaluation in Higher Education*, **14**, 20–31.

Boud D (1992) The use of self-assessment schedules in negotiated learning. *Studies in Higher Education*, **17**, 185–200.

Boud D, Cohen R & Walker D (eds) (1993) *Using Experience for Learning*. The Society for Research into Higher Education and Open University Press, Buckingham.

Boud D, Keogh R & Walker D (1985) *Reflection: Turning Experience into Learning*. Kogan Page, London.

Boud D, Keogh R & Walker D (1996) Promoting reflection in learning: a model. In: *Boundaries of Adult Learning* (eds R Edwards, A Hanson & P Raggatt), pp. 32–56. Routledge, London.

Brookfield SD (1986) *Understanding and Facilitating Adult Learning*. Open University Press, Milton Keynes.

Creek J (2007) The thinking therapist. In: *Contemporary Issues in Occupational Therapy: Reasoning and Reflection* (eds J Creek & A Lawson-Porter), pp. 1–21. John Wiley & Sons, Chichester.

Cross V, Moore A, Morris J, Caladine L, Hilton R & Bristow H (2006) *The Practice Based Educator: A Reflective Tool for CPD and Accreditation*. John Wiley & Sons, Chichester.

Dowie J & Elstein A (eds) (1988) *Professional Judgement: A Reader in Clinical Decision Making*. Cambridge University Press, Cambridge.

Dreyfus H & Dreyfus S (1986) *Mind over Machine: The Power of Human Intuition and Expertise in the Era of the Computer*. Blackwell Publishing Ltd., Oxford.

Eraut M (2002) Editorial. *Learning in Health and Social Care*, **1**(3), 119–121.

Eraut M (2005) Expert and expertise: meanings and perspectives. Editorial. *Learning in Health and Social Care*, **4**(4), 173–179.

Griffin C & Brownhill B (2001) The learning society. In: *The Age of Learning* (ed. P Jarvis), pp. 55-68. Kogan Page, London.

Johns C (2002) *Guided Reflection: Advancing Practice*. Blackwell Science, Oxford.

McNair S (1996) Learner autonomy in a changing world. In: *Boundaries of Adult Learning* (eds R Edwards, A Hanson & P Raggatt), pp. 232–245. Routledge, London.

Megginson D & Whitaker V (2007) *Continuing Professional Development*, 2nd edn. Chartered Institute of Personnel and Development, London.

Schön D (1983) *The Reflective Practitioner: How Professionals Think in Action*. Basic Books, New York.

Watson D (1992) The changing shape of professional education. In: *Developing Professional Education* (eds H Bines & D Watson), pp. 1–10. The Society for Research into Higher Education and Open University Press, Buckingham.

Chapter 6

Learning with others

This chapter addresses:

1. various learning activities that can be pursued in collaboration with others;
2. some of the challenges of undertaking learning projects with others compared with working alone;
3. mechanisms where dialogue with others can assist the learning process.

Introduction

So far, this book has largely focused on lifelong learning and continuing professional development (CPD) as it applies to an individual. This chapter explores the relative merits of learning with other people. Planning and undertaking projects of all kinds in partnership with others can offer significant learning opportunities that are enhanced by dialogue. Learning partnerships can be project oriented and thus time limited. Learning teams may be those that have a common purpose and constantly strive to improve their service for the benefit of users, sometimes through quality assurance mechanisms and sometimes through research activity. On a larger scale, a learning company or learning organisation is an organisation that facilitates the learning of all its employees and seeks to improve and where necessary transform itself and the context in which it operates (Pedlar et al., 1997). A learning company thus assumes active support for learning as well as a collective impetus to learn. These examples reiterate the process of transformation as an outcome of learning. They also acknowledge that learning activity should be actively encouraged through supportive leadership in order that everyone benefits from the learning opportunities that are available, and from the outcome that assumes beneficial change for the community as a whole.

Whilst a learning company has a collective commitment to learning that potentially brings benefits to everyone in the organisation and to the organisation as a whole, on a wider scale there are larger communities where individuals collectively work with their peers to achieve benefits for the whole community. The African philosophy of

Continuing Professional Development in Health and Social Care: Strategies for Lifelong Learning,
Second Edition. Auldeen Alsop.
© 2013 John Wiley & Sons, Ltd. Published 2013 by John Wiley & Sons, Ltd.

Ubuntu denotes connectedness with others and the potential for doing well together and so making a meaningful contribution to the well-being of others (Tutu, 2010). This in turn assists with the development of individuals' capacity for self-realisation but through a sense of belonging and of making an effective contribution to the community as a whole (Kronenberg & Ramugondo, 2011). Communities of learning thrive as the philosophy underpinning them is one of inclusion, so offering support and ways of developing skills, building confidence and thus capacity through the process of collaborative learning.

Although CPD for continued professional registration (or equivalent in different countries) is ultimately a responsibility of the individual, ways of engaging in CPD and lifelong learning activities include collective, collaborative and community activities that may benefit many people as well as contributing to the development of each individual. Each person will engage differently in collaborative projects and thus will record their contribution in a way that reflects their individual learning.

Collaborative learning: projects in partnership

Learning with other people can be a motivating experience as each participant has a responsibility to contribute in order to ensure that expectations of the collaborative venture are met. In partnership, the learning outcomes are likely to be greater for each individual than those that can reasonably be achieved by working alone. Different forms of learning partnerships are possible, from those that casually emerge from the workplace as a support or motivating mechanism for a work-based learning experience, to those that come from like-minded members of a specialist interest group who plan and undertake a project or piece of formal research with a wider remit. Members of multi-professional teams may explore their service together to learn more about costs, benefits, shortcomings and positive achievements. More formal collaborative partnerships can be formed for research purposes, potentially but not exclusively for participatory action research (Kemmis & McTaggart, 2000). On a wider scale, uni- or multi-professional international collaborations can form to support global projects around practice, research, education and publication using various technological means of communication.

A partnership of two or more like-minded people with a common professional development interest or goal becomes a collaboration that can lead to significant learning. A journal club would be an example. A partnership between a student and supervisor or between a clinician and mentor can offer learning experiences for both partners. Sometimes the collaborations have learning as a prime target. For example, a simple investigation, formal or informal, of an agreed phenomenon or set of circumstances can result in learning and a new understanding of the relative merits of a practice for all those involved. A collaborative project established purposely to explore or set up a new service may have different primary goals but can also result in learning. A formal collaborative research project with a clear research question and aims will provide a learning venture based on a search for evidence that may also lead to changes in practice and benefits to service users. Collaborative enquiry is claimed to be one of the keys to organisational learning in that learning takes place between people 'in a relationship of persons acting collaboratively' where the outcomes of learning 'cannot be fully measured in terms of what individuals take away, but by the new meaning which is created together' (Pedlar et al., 1997). Other collaborative learning can take place between students and/or practitioners, within local groups such as specialist interest groups, or through service learning initiatives (Lorenzo et al., 2006; Healey, 2011; Pollard & Parks, 2011; see also Chapter 10). Many of these situations have transformational outcomes for participants. Ways of collaborating and learning through action learning sets are discussed in Chapter 12. Again, collaboration need not be hindered by distance and international time frames. New technology presents many ways of communicating that allow participation from interested parties at local, national or international venues.

Longer term projects, as referred to earlier, bring both challenges and rewards. Many of them are set up for significant periods of time, often months, and sometimes a few years, that may test the tolerance of some group members. These projects require longer term commitment from the team membership. As with all projects, tolerance of different opinions, some give-and-take in the decision-making process, reliance on members completing allocated tasks within an allotted timeframe and trust that everyone is working towards goals that are commonly agreed and understood are prerequisites to success. In the long run, the rewards are also shared.

Collaborative ventures can be exciting as several people often from different backgrounds address a common issue or project bringing many different perspectives and much useful knowledge to the venture. However, there can also be challenges when working in partnership as there can be many different personalities amongst the group. Some people may not be team players and will try to dominate or disrupt proceedings in their own way. Clearly, it is not beneficial to the group to have to manage dominant people as it puts the project at risk. Different views are welcome but eventually there has to be consensus amongst the group members about ways forward. One way of addressing the issue is to agree at the outset a set of ground rules that operate for the duration of the project. The group must have a designated project manager who ultimately takes decisions and keeps the project on track. Ground rules must also include respect for others' views even though a suggestion may not be used. However, instead of using a group there may be times when 'going it alone' is actually a favoured option rather than a collaboration or operating a consensus model. Time may be at a premium and one focused person may be all that is required to undertake the project and complete the task. However, working alone can be somewhat isolating, so being able to draw on support from colleagues as required can be a helpful option. Contact with others at a social level either in person or through social media online can minimise feelings of working in isolation.

Learning events

Some collective learning events are on a much smaller scale. For example, a team awayday offers the opportunity to explore a common issue; a study day can provide avenues for critically examining a specific topic; a conference may draw on different perspectives on new policy or procedures and enlighten the audience; a workshop or residential weekend can offer a more focused opportunity to generate ideas for a project and a plan of action. These opportunities bring like-minded people together to explore issues and perspectives on a common goal and to generate new ideas or ways forward. Projects involving widespread involvement of different stakeholders who have a vested interest in the project have their roots in Whole Systems Thinking or Whole Systems Development initiatives (Pedlar et al., 1997). These events can involve a large number of people, groups of whom proportionately represent their peers in offering their views on the proposed project. All such learning events bring people together, not only where there is a common purpose to achieve an agreed outcome but also as an opportunity for gaining new insights into the topic and the strengths and perspectives of members of the group. A collaborative venture can also offer an opportunity for extending each individual's knowledge and skills.

Participatory action research

Participatory action research is a formalised way of undertaking research in partnership with others, often in relation to an aspect of their practice that is not only common to the researchers but also problematic to them. According to Kemmis and McTaggart (2000) the fundamental idea of action learning is about bringing people together to learn from each other's experience. This form of research can thus be used by service users and practitioners working collaboratively in an area of practice where there is a common issue to explore and potentially resolve. This type of research occurs commonly in situations where people want to make changes thoughtfully after some relevant critical reflection on what occurs. What actually occurs has first to be discovered by searching not only for familiar practices but also for those practices that are unfamiliar, unseen or unnoticed, and unmasking them to make the 'unfamiliar familiar' (Kemmis & McTaggart, 2000). The research involves uncovering and then questioning assumptions. It is a cyclical process comprising four stages: (1) planning, (2) action, (3) observation of the impact of the action and then (4) reflection on the action and its impact (Kramer-Roy, 2011). The learning occurs both individually and collectively and is said to be emancipatory for those who participate as it empowers participants to create change in their social circumstances. According to Kemmis and McTaggart (2000, p. 597), participatory action research is a form of learning with others by 'doing', so enabling people to be released from 'the constraints of irrational, unproductive, unjust and unsatisfying social structures that limit self-development and self-determination' (see Kramer-Roy, 2011 and Bryant et al., 2011 for examples of participatory action research in health and social care settings).

Storytelling

One activity that may assist learning is the opportunity to tell and listen to stories. Storytelling has a long history as a way in which humans communicate, share information with and entertain people. Storytelling should be distinguished from the expression of opinions (which tend to lack a plot) and reports that provide factual accounts but without meaning. Stories offer facts-as-experience as told and inter- preted by a raconteur and they are enriched by being infused with meaning with which a listener can engage (Gabriel, 2000). Stories have key features that make each recognisable as a story. These include a setting, characters, an initiating event, some effort to attain a goal, a consequence, a reaction and a resolution (McAdams, 1993). As McAdams suggests, the story is a natural package for organising information. Stories have both an entertaining and enlightening effect. They can arouse emotions and prompt interpretation so that meaning is attributed to them. Figure 6.1 presents a true story of a developing friendship that led to the coining of a new phrase, that of 'critical kinship', which is described later. The key features of a story as identified by McAdams can be recognised in this story.

As a learning activity, storytelling may be delivered in such a way that the essence of the story becomes memorable and meaningful and may bring new insights that could impact on practice. Whilst, for example, presentations at conferences can be informative, stories that are told more informally to an audience can become engaging and provide the impetus to think more critically about practice. Stories are products of personal experience. Telling and listening to stories assist individuals to make sense of the world. The result may lead to changes that have a lasting effect within the professional world.

Abma (1999) explored the role of storytelling in a therapeutic context. Citing Forester (1993), Abma illustrated how stories about real incidents in practice could play a powerful role in transforming practice by working as a mirror and highlighting discrepancies between intentions and behaviour. Any ambiguity in stories could thus prompt reflection on experiences and open up opportunities for further discourse and potential change. In some ways, storytelling may be no more than informal conversations about unusual incidents in practice. Active listening and questioning as stories are told can raise issues for further investigation, debate and possible resolution, all with the ultimate intention of learning. Case stories presented to an audience that can engage and critically consider possible avenues to resolve the challenges can add to a practitioner's repertoire of scenarios for later reference. Similarly, critical incidents recounted as stories can be explored. These tend to require more systematic investigation, much of which can be done through conversation, reflection and critical examination of particular practices that may ultimately require modification.

Mechanisms for supporting learning

Supervision is a common support mechanism used in large organisations delivering health and social care. A named supervisor in professional practice would normally oversee the professional development of junior practitioners, helping them to grow in their role, feel more confident in practice and develop their knowledge and skills for enhancing their career prospects. A regular appraisal or performance review with a supervisor should formalise any intentions with regard to CPD for addressing

Our journey started when the two of us who come from quite different backgrounds and professional lives were brought together by chance, initially through a distant working relationship that centred on learning. We subsequently became travelling companions in both a physical and metaphorical sense. Our journey became the medium for sharing our experiences and gaining critical insights into each other's world. Initially, train journeys taken together provided opportunities for conversations, which were engaging and somewhat exploratory about each other's academic interests and ideas. Over time, the one to one conversations gathered momentum and led to more serious philosophical debates. Conversations included some 'checking out' unconsciously then more consciously of detail as specific areas of interest were discussed. The shared agenda led to revelations that affirmed shared knowledge, values and an interest in research. Eventually, deeper conversations took place that entailed critical discussion and reflection on such topics as biographical research, narrative and personal involvement with specific research topics and agenda. So the metaphorical journey evolved.

Our conversations became absorbing, personally revealing and more meaningful, with more concentrated critical discussion and debate that focused on complex issues of shared interest and concern. There was more commitment to sharing and revealing personal strengths and limitations as mutual trust developed. Intellectual critical conversations brought momentum and their own rewards as our personal need for higher-level academic challenge, not otherwise available through day-to-day vocational/occupational activities, began to be met. Reflection on the various conversations continued alone after each rail journey and allowed opportunity for each of us to develop understanding and personal sense-making. The combined challenge of critical conversation and debate based on a shared agenda, yet stimulated by exposure to different perspectives within what was perceived to be a 'safe' partnership, helped us to develop new insights and promoted our personal confidence and intellectual growth. Personal reflection both within and external to the relationship strengthened our commitment to the collaboration. Learning to share critical ideas not only strengthened our relationship but promoted our personal and professional growth.

One train journey was particularly memorable. Zoë misquoted a phrase from Paulo Freire's preface to Peter McLaren's book *Critical Pedagogy* (1995). The actual phrase in the book's preface cited 'intellectual kinship'. However, in our conversation the term 'kinship' was somehow elided with the title of the book to create the new idea of 'critical kinship'. We came to realise that a different phrase had been coined through a process of creative, serendipitous reworking of memory to produce something new from familiar fragments. The new phrase really appealed to us. As we reflected on it, the term began to take on a particular meaning. The separate meanings of each of the two words within the phrase combined to portray the relationship that had been emerging between us. The sharper intellectual connotations of the word 'critical' and the warmer more human resonance of the word 'kinship' clearly described the intellectual yet mutually supportive state of our relationship.

This critical aspect was key for us as we questioned our assumptions and preconceptions and shared our ideas. It was invaluable to have established enough of a connection to trust each other so that we could engage willingly to resolve any inconsistencies yet still respect any remaining differences.

What we have come to understand by critical kinship is the relationship between two people who are working along the same lines but whose different perspectives and experiences can be used to unpack, challenge and critique each other's assumptions and tacit theorising. This ability to be 'critical' comes from a position of trustful respect and understanding which offers the 'kinship'. This means that we each feel safe enough with the other person to hear the questions without feeling defensive or undermined. The mutuality of the relationship reflects the democratic approach at the heart of action research and enables us to exist in the balanced power relationship of critical kinship.

Zoë Parker and Auldeen Alsop, 2010

Figure 6.1   A journey to critical kinship

gaps in knowledge and skills. Discussions in supervision sessions might also include suggestions about CPD activities that might go some way towards meeting career aspirations. A supervisor might facilitate visits, secondments or other relevant experiences to aid professional development. The supervisee would be responsible for following through the suggestions for development and for reporting outcomes back to the supervisor. Records of the CPD should be kept in a learning log or portfolio.

Mentorship, also addressed elsewhere in this book, is another common strategy for supporting professionals in their role and for encouraging forms of professional development that might support a wider strategy for career development. A mentor is normally a person sought specifically for their experience in practice, management or research who can offer advice to the mentee on dealing with situations that arise in their field of work. A mentor is likely to be someone working outside of the department or organisation in which the mentee operates. This helps with objectivity in addressing issues of concern or where guidance is sought. Together the mentor and mentee may decide on a course of action to be taken to address any work-related issues. CPD strategies can also be discussed to assist the mentee in developing knowledge and skills for career development.

Critical companionship and the role of a critical companion have come from the nursing literature and research (Titchen, 1998). Critical companionship was coined as a strategy for personal and professional development using a critical companion or facilitator to promote learning. It was intended as a person-centred strategy for helping practitioners to understand the nature of their professional knowledge base, to create new professional craft knowledge from their practice and to shape their new knowledge and practice. The critical companion is considered to be an experienced facilitator who accompanies a practitioner on an experiential learning journey by helping to bring to consciousness issues arising from specific situations for critical review. New professional craft knowledge can then be created. A person-centred approach to facilitating learning is used that includes articulation of the processes and strategies involved (Titchen et al., 2004). There may be benefits to using this model within the health and social care professions.

Critical kinship is proposed here as a relationship rooted in a shared sense of purpose for praxis. As two people engage in a dynamic dialogue that becomes a mutually educative process and where benefits are quickly apparent, there is potential for a more meaningful relationship to develop. The dialogue brings affirmation of values and enhances both personal and collaborative endeavour. What emerges is a sustainable relationship as a medium for learning and personal growth. The 'critical' aspect of the relationship offers critique, debate, challenge and change. The 'kinship' fosters empathy, understanding, trust and respect. The emergence of the concept of critical kinship is recounted as a true story in Figure 6.1. Critical kinship is thus experienced as a deep meaningful relationship that supports and enhances personal and professional development.

Social spaces

The story of the emergence of the term 'critical kinship' (Figure 6.1) shows that new insights can emerge from conversations in all sorts of social spaces including trains.

Therefore, it could be suggested that learning can take place at any time and anywhere provided that the mind and senses are open to exploration and to engaging critically in experiences or new ways of thinking about practices. Some important conversations take place in social spaces such as in the coffee room or over lunch in the local cafe, while chatting informally in a queue or walking with a colleague between different locations. These may not start off as deep and meaningful conversations, yet some observation from one person may trigger thoughts that lead to more serious exchanges, perhaps as reflections on events that shed light on some aspect of professional work. Ideas may be generated that lead to more focused learning conversations or events. Accommodation at places of work is often at a premium and social spaces set aside for staff breaks are not always given priority, yet when available they can be fruitful learning spaces. Chance or even planned encounters in any social space away from a work desk can free the mind momentarily from the pressure of work-related tasks and offer space for conversations that can be either reflective or creative and lead to bigger learning projects. These chance, yet meaningful conversations, may be worth noting in a learning log. One such new learning project might be writing up a shared learning experience, including its application to practice, for publication.

Publication

One project where distinct choices about partnership have to be made is when writing for publication. It is easy to think of publication more as a process of dissemination of information than a process of learning, but learning features widely. Shared effort brings shared rewards and collaboration in publishing is often a preferred choice when it comes to writing an article for a refereed journal or writing a book for publication.

Articles can have a single or multiple authors. If the article is based on research it not unusual for several authors involved in the original research to make a contribution to the article. The lead author is the first named author on the published article. He or she is normally the person with whom the journal editor communicates and whose contact details are provided in the publication. There are time challenges with multiple authors as each version of the article may need to be commented on by each author and any changes agreed on. There may also be differences in viewpoints that have to be managed. Various versions of an article can be in circulation so identifying the number of each draft version is crucial to ensure that the most up-to-date version is reviewed. Single authorship offers more control over preparation of an article and it can speed up the process. Colleagues may be prepared to give feedback on early drafts but the decision about what is submitted to the journal editor rests with the author. Preparing an article for publication requires considerable research to ensure a sound basis for the work and also attention to detail with regard to the preparation of the script in accordance with the authors' guidelines, as applicable to the chosen journal. Further work is often required once reviews of the article are received. Additional reading and/or research may be required to ascertain the relevant information required by reviewers. It is always worthwhile to ensure that the article demonstrates the relevance to service users of the research or other key information presented. In total, the work involved can be onerous but once published, the article provides great evidence of the research for CPD purposes.

Preparation of a book for publication is a longer term project. A book can be written by a single author, several authors or by one or more people who act as editors. In this case, chapters are written by individuals, often experts in their particular field. Each model presents its own challenges in terms of preparation of the chapters within a given time, ensuring collectively that chapters come together as a book. Where there are several contributors, the authors may write in different styles, there may be gaps, omissions or duplication of material. Editors must deal with this and it is a very time-consuming activity. In this model, chapters can be written simultaneously but time is often needed to deal with the editing process of bringing individual chapters together as a book. In contrast, there are time issues for a single author who researches and writes each chapter. The aid of a colleague to offer feedback on work is very welcome. Two or more authors can write chapters separately or together, first ensuring that their writing styles are compatible and there is agreement about who is lead author. Planning, researching material to support the writing and the preparation of chapters is a shared activity. Shared authorship immediately brings support for the process of preparing the script for publication. The benefits of shared authorship are also shared, but on publication of the book each author can produce evidence of CPD. Anyone who writes a chapter for an edited book can similarly produce evidence of CPD.

Summary

This chapter has suggested that learning with other people can be beneficial, providing welcome support for individual learners and wider knowledge to the group as projects are undertaken collaboratively. Groups of people bring different perspectives as individuals contribute in different ways and use their unique strengths to support the project as a whole. Groups of people can comprise one or two individuals working together on a project to work-based teams, larger companies and, more globally, to wider communities who learn and benefit collectively from the collaboration. All individuals who participate with others in an initiative can gain experience and learn from making their contribution and from engaging with the contributions of others. Projects such as evaluations of practice and research projects can also bring significant benefits to service users, as can attendance at conferences and study days that prompt reflection on, and improvements in practice. Reflection and dialogue about projects are important to ensure learning and to consider change in practice. Telling and listening to stories can also offer collective learning opportunities as tales of events are recounted that resonate with participants and prompt reflection on their own practice. Various support mechanisms for learning are also considered in this chapter. Reflection on events and discussion in a one-to-one relationship with a colleague about ways of moving forward in practice can help clarify issues of concern and boost confidence. All incidents of learning with others potentially serve to enhance knowledge and improve practice for service users. Records in CPD logs should reflect a variety of ways in which learning with others has made a contribution to personal learning and professional development.

References

Abma T (1999) Powerful stories: the role of stories in sustaining and transforming professional practice within a mental hospital. In: *Making Meaning of Narratives* (eds R Josselson & A Lieblich), pp. 169–196. Sage Publications, Thousand Oaks, CA.

Bryant W, McKay E, Beresford P & Vacher G (2011) An occupational perspective on participatory action research. In: *Occupational Therapies with Borders*, Vol. **2** (eds F Kronenberg, N Pollard & D Sakellariou), pp. 367–374. Elsevier, Edinburgh.

Forester J (1993) Learning from practice stories. In: *The Argumentative Turn in Policy Analysis and Planning* (eds F Fisher & J Forester), pp. 186–209. UCL Press, London.

Freire P (1995) Preface. In: *Critical Pedagogy a Predatory Culture: Oppositional Politics in a Post-modern Era* (ed. P McLaren), pp. ix–xi. Routledge, New York.

Gabriel Y (2000) *Storytelling in Organisations: Facts, Fictions and Fantasies*. Oxford University Press, Oxford.

Healey J (2011) Empowering learning environments for developing occupational therapy practice in the UK. In: *Occupational Therapies without Borders*, Vol. **2** (eds F Kronenberg, N Pollard & D Sakellariou), pp. 305–312. Churchill Livingstone, Edinburgh.

Kemmis S & McTaggart R (2000) Participatory action research. In: *Handbook of Qualitative Research* (eds NK Denzin & YS Lincoln), 2nd edn, pp. 567–606. Sage Publications, Thousand Oaks, CA.

Kramer-Roy D (2011) Occupational injustice in Pakistani families with disabled children in the UK: a PAR study. In: *Occupational Therapies without Borders*, Vol. **2** (eds F Kronenberg, N Pollard & D Sakellariou), pp. 375–384. Churchill Livingstone, Edinburgh.

Kronenberg F & Ramugondo E (2011) Ubuntourism: engaging divided people in post-aparteid South Africa. In: *Occupational Therapies without Borders*, Vol. **2** (eds F Kronenberg, N Pollard & D Sakellariou), pp. 195–208. Churchill Livingstone, Edinburgh.

Lorenzo T, Duncan M, Buchanan H & Alsop A (eds) (2006) *Practice and Service Learning in Occupational Therapy*. John Wiley & Sons, Chichester.

McAdams DP (1993) *The Stories We Live By: Personal Myths and the Making of Self*. Guilford Press, New York.

Pedlar M, Burgogne J & Boydell T (1997) *The Learning Company, a Strategy for Sustainable Development*, 2nd edn. McGraw-Hill, London.

Pollard N & Parks S (2011) Community publishing: occupational therapy narratives and 'local publics'. In: *Occupational Therapies without Borders*, Vol. **2** (eds F Kronenberg, N Pollard & D Sakellariou), pp. 171–178. Churchill Livingstone, Edinburgh.

Titchen A (1998) *Professional craft knowledge and patient-centred nursing and the facilitation of its development*. Unpublished PhD thesis, Oxford University.

Titchen A, McGinley M & McCormack B (2004) Blending self-knowledge and professional knowledge in person-centred care. In: *Developing Practice Knowledge for Health Professionals* (eds J Higgs, B Richardson & M Abrandt Dahlgren), pp. 107–126. Butterworth-Heinemann, Oxford.

Tutu D (2010) Foreword. In: *(2011) Occupational Therapies without Borders*, Vol. **2** (eds F Kronenberg, N Pollard & D Sakellariou), p. ix. Churchill Livingstone, Edinburgh.

Chapter 7

Learning in the workplace

This chapter addresses:

1. various formal and non-formal ways in which learning can be undertaken in the workplace and the nature of experiential learning;
2. the responsibility of practitioners to use learning to transform practice;
3. organisational issues that impact on learning in the workplace.

Introduction

Most therapists and students of the health and social care professions would argue that the workplace provides one of the most meaningful settings for learning about professional practice. The workplace offers the opportunity for the learner to watch professional colleagues at work, participate in a full range of professional practices and related discussions, and gain insight and experience of operating within the real context of practice, with all its challenges. Learning in the workplace has previously related largely to 'placements' associated with pre-registration learning. Now employees are said to be extending their educational capabilities through their work, so helping to transform that work by creating new work practices and improvements within the organisation (Boud & Garrick, 1999). Jarvis (2001) also recognised that knowledge was growing at an exponential rate creating a demand for continuing learning opportunities within the workplace. Work has been promoted as providing continual and often complex challenges in knowledge and skill application so prompting personal, professional and organisational development (Rounce & Workman, 2005).

Continuing Professional Development in Health and Social Care: Strategies for Lifelong Learning,
Second Edition. Auldeen Alsop.
© 2013 John Wiley & Sons, Ltd. Published 2013 by John Wiley & Sons, Ltd.

Lemanski et al. (2011) attempted to categorise work-based learning, recognising the growing interest in learning in the workplace not only in the United Kingdom but also across Europe. Three types of learning were cited:

1. *Learning for work* – such as work experience/placements.
2. *Learning at work* – such as programmes arranged and supported by the organisation (often not assessed).
3. *Learning through work* – such as on-site courses that are formally assessed and accredited.

Some work-based projects are undertaken in collaboration with staff in a university. Post-registration students engaging in such projects learn from both their peers at university and the community of practice within the organisation to which they relate. A useful definition of work-based learning for this chapter emerged from Clarke and Copeland (2003) and was cited by Lemanski et al. (2011, p. 8):

> Work-based learning is commonly taken to refer to structured learning opportunities which derive from, or which are focused on, the work role of individuals within organisations (Clarke & Copeland, 2003).

This is a helpful definition that embraces all three types of learning in the workplace. However, the three examples of work-based learning for a particular purpose relate to more structured learning experiences that are pre-defined for learners, often to promote their personal and professional development within a particular environment. Another example of workplace learning, which is not pre-defined, is experiential learning.

Experiential learning

Health and social care professionals will normally be well versed in reflective practice (Schön, 1983) and experiential learning (Kolb, 1984). Here, learning is not necessarily pre-planned but prompted by unique events in the workplace that actively engage the mind and senses of the practitioner. The underlying theory of experiential learning stems from the belief that learning emerges from an individual's engagement with selected situations and actively reflecting on them after the event. Reflection-on-action (Schön, 1983) is a dynamic process that involves bringing back to mind the events that occurred, exploring them through a conversation with self or with others and critically examining them to determine what happened, what could have happened and whether the outcome could have been different. Triggers for reflection might include problems or disturbances to the normal routine or other stimuli emerging from questioning practice either alone or with colleagues (Kember, 2001). Johns (2002) commented that reflection helped develop an understanding of contradictions in practice, for example, between desirable and actual practice. Reflection on practice is seen as integral to learning through preceptorship schemes as more formalised schemes of learning established for newly qualified practitioners (Morley, 2007).

Those reflecting on an experience in the workplace might consider the following:

- What went well?
- What did not go so well?
- What, if anything, could have been done differently?
- What have been the reactions of others to this event?
- What have I learned from what I have done, seen, heard and considered?
- What steps do I need to take to understand the situation further (conversations, research, reading)?
- How will this affect my future practice?

In addition, the importance of articulating practice knowledge is key to the process of scrutinising the rationale for choices and decisions in practice. Engaging peers in critical conversations about practice helps establish the reasoning processes that occurred to inform decisions and thus the consequences of actions (Richardson et al., 2004). Engaging honestly and systematically with questions about events in practice should help make explicit the learning that occurred. Boud et al. (1985) have suggested that reflection-on-action is the key to learning from experience. Those who are more likely to engage in reflection-on-action are those whose skills in self-directed learning are already reasonably well developed as they have the motivation to learn and are open, not only to learning opportunities, but also to ambiguities in practice and others' points of view.

Formal and non-formal learning in the workplace

From the above brief overview, different forms of workplace learning have been introduced. However, Breen (2005) considers these as formal and non-formal learning experiences and examines some of the issues involved. Breen (2005) suggested that work-related learning could occur in formal or non-formal contexts. Formal learning tends to have a structured curriculum that is devised and administered by others and that leads to some recognised award. However, success might depend on the potential for finding learning activities in the workplace that are relevant to the curriculum. This could be challenging. Billett (1999) pointed out that experiences in the workplace are dictated by the organisation's goals and activities and not by academic expectations. Where formal learning does occur, it tends to benefit the individual rather than the organisation, and so it may not necessarily be supported by the organisation. Non-formal learning, on the other hand, does not have the structure of a curriculum but may contribute to organisational performance more effectively than formal learning initiatives. Planned non-formal learning opportunities would normally be made relevant to an individual's personal goals as well as to the goals of the organisation. It should lead to enhanced personalised knowledge. Ongoing learning through active engagement in novel situations in the workplace can instil confidence and enable personal and professional growth. Effective work-based learning supports the lifelong learning agenda as it can also be relevant to the wider context of life. According to Billett (1999), knowledge secured in the workplace is likely to be different from that acquired in an academic environment because the knowledge-constructing experiences are different. Also, the activities in which individuals engage in the workplace influence the knowledge that is constructed. Real-life learning experiences can occur for practitioners irrespective of the stage of their professional development.

Government papers have often supported the notion of work-based learning, particularly in relation to learning to implement new policies and initiatives in health and social care. Many opportunities can be seized to promote professional development at the same time as allowing engagement in, and the development of, service-based initiatives. However, maximising the effects of learning in the workplace will depend on the extent of the employee's active engagement in service delivery and on personal reflection on the practices that occur. This includes reflection on the options that are presented, the decisions that are taken and the alternatives that are rejected, and the rationale for these decisions. New learning will only occur if the learning strategy includes reflection on all relevant experiences.

Formal learning

Learning in the workplace can be formalised in several ways. Formally approved research undertaken with colleagues or alone can not only lead to personal and organisational learning, but can also shape future practice in a much wider sense. Learning through project work, where goals, aims and a timeframe are specifically set, can also lead to positive change in service provision and outcomes for service users. Some projects may emerge from discussions in an individual appraisal or performance review. Ideas for projects may be put forward by an individual or the line manager and may be supported within the service where there are potential gains for the service and service users. Other projects may emerge from uni- or multi-disciplinary team discussions and be undertaken collaboratively with colleagues to improve service efficiency, effectiveness or both. Any such work-based project will thus offer learning opportunities for individuals, and possibly for teams and the wider organisation or profession. At an individual level, organisations may support individuals in pursuing recognised education awards that are undertaken in the workplace, particularly if the activities or qualifications undertaken are likely to enhance service provision. National Vocational Qualifications in the United Kingdom offer learners the chance to develop skills directly related to their employment. Local colleges and universities or other external accredited bodies may provide distance learning materials or e-learning opportunities to support learning in the workplace. Individuals may pursue recognised academic awards in this way up to doctoral level.

Colleges and institutions of higher education are now finding very creative ways of promoting learning in the workplace, recognising that health and social care professionals may not readily be able to take time out of practice to study. The need for ongoing learning and professional development of individuals may be dictated to some extent by their regulatory body and its expectations of updating of practice knowledge, continuous learning and improvement. However, many full-time employees are likely to find it very difficult to take time out of practice to fulfil the expectation. Benefit may derive from such schemes as 'CPD Anywhere' (www.shu.ac.uk/faculties/hwb/cpd/anywhere), which is a resource and support framework developed especially for health care professionals that allows them to choose the time, pace and place of delivery of the learning opportunity. Individuals who sign up to the scheme gain access to an e-portfolio for recording learning activities and can study topics of their choice that are current to practice. These are formally presented e-learning strategies about current issues pertinent to practice as they link to a higher education system. However, they may not necessarily contribute to learning for a higher degree as there may be no mode of assessment or confirmation of learning. Alternatively, more formal schemes such as accreditation of prior learning (APL) may be operated by the university allowing individuals to seek academic credit for their learning in the workplace.

All these strategies support the notion of lifelong learning and can be personalised to meet individual needs and goals. There will be costs associated with certificated learning and the responsibility for payment of fees will need to be negotiated locally. Organisations may support their personnel in undertaking formal courses if the outcome is likely to be of benefit to the service. Health care professionals can obtain significant guidance and support from their professional body with regard to strategies and opportunities for professional development. Reference to the relevant website will provide information on specific courses and qualifications for advancing practice and those for continuing professional development (CPD) to meet Health and Care Professions Council (HCPC) or other regulatory body requirements.

Informal learning

Marsick and Watkins (1990) theorised that informal and incidental learning in the workplace were not the same, the key distinction being that informal learning was defined as intentional whereas incidental learning was not. Garrick (1999, p. 219) argued that the distinction was dubious, suggesting that 'accidental' learning better described 'a spontaneous, contingent form of learning where something fruitful or transformative happens without deliberation'. When the totally unexpected happens, the full extent of its significance for learning may not be appreciated until sometime later.

For the purpose of this chapter, informal learning can be thought of as learning that is not pre-planned but may occur unexpectedly at any time and any place. Experiences, in order to be transformed into learning, must be examined critically as described earlier in order that the new knowledge can be identified. Garrick (1999, p. 227) contended that it was the non-routine circumstances that force professionals 'into the kind of reflective thinking that changes beliefs, values and assumptions'. Not all experiences will thus offer learning opportunities but selected non-routine experiences may prove quite significant in adding to learning.

Social workers

Social workers in England have their own approved scheme for CPD outlined in The Post-qualifying Framework for Social Work Education and Training (General Social Care Council, 2005). The framework:

- stresses the need for user and carer involvement in education and training;
- relates specifically to National Occupational Standards for Social Work;
- is based on the principle that academic and professional learning be fully integrated;
- focuses on the assessment of competence in practice;
- advocates inter-professional education.

Social workers who, until August 2012, were regulated by the General Social Care Council are now regulated by the HCPC. The transition of all functions from one council to another may take time to achieve but it is known that social workers will eventually have to fulfil the same criteria for CPD as those professions already regulated by the HCPC. Following the change of regulation, the ethos of the profession will remain much the same. However, at the time of writing it is not currently clear what the eventual status of the post-qualifying framework will be, although it may still serve as a guide to CPD for the profession. Work-based learning is still likely to be the preferred mode of learning that allows other essential criteria, such as the involvement of service users and carers, to be met. Formal learning through approved university modules and courses that can be undertaken as practice-based learning modules is expected to form the basis of much of the profession's CPD.

Accredited learning in the workplace

Increasingly, universities have come to acknowledge the value of learning in the workplace and its place in developing (or further developing) knowledge and skills that are worthy of academic reward. Post-qualification awards, such as Master's degrees, can include modules that have been purposely approved for work-based learning. Modules may have learning outcomes that are defined in general terms and then interpreted more specifically by the learner. For example, someone undertaking an MSc in Care of Older People might be required to critically explore the potential costs, benefits and take-up of defined physical activities as available in the local setting. The module has general expectations but the student addresses them specifically in the context of his or her work environment. Other modules may be labelled Independent Studies. In this case, the learner negotiates with the tutor the individual learning outcomes that he or she wishes to achieve through independent learning in the workplace. These learning outcomes will be agreed as being achievable in the workplace in the given timeframe and sufficiently academic to warrant Master's level credit towards the overall award. The topic of the study could be unique to the individual learner but approval would depend on satisfying any ethical considerations related to the study. The work that is undertaken for any module will need to be assessed formally in accordance with the regulations of the awarding institution.

Modules of this kind offer academic freedom to pursue studies of specific interest to the individual and that potentially may also benefit the service in which he or she works. Similarly, over the past 10 years or more, professional doctorates have emerged as an option for busy professionals who wish to gain an academic award at doctoral level. Both the United States and Australia were awarding professional doctorates before the United Kingdom (Rounce et al., 2005). A definition of a professional doctorate has been put forward by the UK Council for Graduate Education as follows:

> A professional doctorate is a programme of advanced study and research which, whilst satisfying the University criteria for the award of a doctorate, is designed to meet the specific needs of a professional group external to the University, and which develops the capability of individuals to work within a professional context (UK Council for Graduate Education, 2002, p. 62).

Professional doctorates, rooted as they are in professional practice, tend to be more structured than PhDs, which are wholly research based. Professional doctorates and PhDs place different, but equal, demands on the learner/researcher. Professional doctorates are normally available on a part-time basis and offer a set programme of high-level academic studies to small groups of people often from mixed professional backgrounds. The early stages of the programme may be modular in format. Initially the focus will be on the development of knowledge and skills in research techniques as preparation for an individual research study at the end of the programme. In contrast, the PhD is wholly research based. The student is allocated a Director of Studies by the university and one or two other experts who together make up the supervisory team. The student meets regularly with the team and sometimes with individual supervisors. The team guides the student through university expectations with regard to regulations, protocol, ethical approval and study regime and advises on the research but the majority of the work is self-directed by the student. Any research undertaken within a health or social care context will be subject to the research ethics procedures of that organisation as well as the university ethics procedures. It is the student's responsibility to establish current procedures for ethics approval.

Conflicts of interest

Workplace learning can make conflicting demands on the learner because of his or her dual role as service provider and learner (Ramage, 2005). Good mentorship can assist with disentangling the responsibilities of the two roles and assessing the outcome for each one. The learning tasks may be part of a set curriculum. They may be related to addressing specific goals in a personal learning contract. Learning may also derive from unanticipated learning opportunities. Whichever is appropriate, the learning is still likely to be experiential and require careful analysis and reflection on outcomes. Only then can conflicting demands be identified, addressed and resolved. Organisations that support work-based learning should understand the conflicts associated with the employee as learner. If the learning is to be derived from projects set by the organisation, for example, an assessment of the potential of a new service, then conflicts should be minimal. The project investigations should be undertaken with integrity and with full consideration of the potential impact of the proposal, particularly on staff, and should be unbiased. The experience of undertaking the project will benefit the individual project worker, particularly in the development of project management skills. The project findings, presented orally or in a report, will be of benefit to the organisation.

If the learning task is set by an educational establishment then normally the learner would first discuss and agree the task with a line manager who hopefully would support the project and enable the employee to complete the work. However, there may still be conflicts of interest that need to be addressed. The educational establishment will set the agenda for the work-based learning project, but the method of completing it may need to be negotiated in the workplace. However, the university will expect the assessment to be completed by the learner. Unless otherwise agreed, the assessment is normally personal to the individual submitting it. No other person, even from the employing organisation, is necessarily entitled to see it. Anyone undertaking work-based learning as part of an educational course should therefore clarify and agree expectations with the educational institution and the line manager before undertaking the work.

How to make the most of workplace learning

The workplace provides such a rich source of learning material that opportunities for ongoing learning and professional development should be plentiful. Taking up some opportunities may need negotiation within the workplace but others should be readily available as part of everyday practice. Those employees who have contracts that provide for rotations between different departments within an organisation will have a new source of learning every time the rotation takes place. These experiences will normally be available to practitioners to help consolidate learning, to give the practitioner further insights into different areas of practice and to help the practitioner decide on a preferred area of practice in which to specialise later in a career.

Making the most of experiences that occur naturally in everyday practice is dependent on the employee being alert to situations that provide opportunities for new learning. Even though some practice on a daily basis may be fairly routine, every now and again an unusual case will require different solutions to the norm, so making the routine situation into a new learning experience. Compared with most routine situations, these non-routine occurrences are more likely to demand more of what Schön (1983) labels 'reflection-in-action' and novel interventions that address the problem in hand. These cases provide key workplace learning experiences for later 'reflection-on-action' and analysis. The new learning should be documented in a portfolio in such a way that it is ready for presentation to the regulatory body to demonstrate CPD. Any supplementary activities, such as exploring related research, gaining more information on a diagnosis, reading related articles, will provide supplementary information that can also be documented in précis form, but in such a way that the new learning is highlighted.

Not only does the immediate work environment provide opportunities, so do other environments within the same organisation or in other organisations. For example, it may be possible to negotiate entry to a different location to work in a different clinical or non-clinical specialty for a fixed period of time. Different departments not only offer different learning experiences, but also enhance working relationships between departments within an organisation.

Shadowing experts in different locations provides similar opportunities for learning. Shadowing may be negotiated within the employing authority or in another organisation. Even short visits to different settings can offer real learning experiences that can be reflected upon and evaluated for any new knowledge or skills that have emerged from the experience. Colleagues who work in similar specialty areas in different organisations may wish to host a visit to each other's organisation to share good practice or develop ideas for improving practice. Making the most of planned experiences entails good preparation before the visit as well as an overall evaluation after the experience. For example, thinking about the visit beforehand can lead to the formulation of a number of questions that could be posed during the visit. Setting down goals and aims of the visit can focus the mind on achieving a good outcome. Knowing what it is that you want to gain from the visit, and sharing that information with the host, will assist the host in planning the best use of time and targeting access to the people or physical resources that will be most helpful. Personal reflection on the various aspects of the visit (including the preparations) should highlight strengths and limitations of, and the benefits accrued from, the visit. Reflection should also highlight the next steps to be taken in continuing learning or in order to follow up on gaps in knowledge that the visit has exposed. Offering to share the experience with colleagues after the event can help. A lunchtime seminar or other informal meeting may provide the opportunity to discuss issues emerging from the visit with colleagues. In particular, it is worth highlighting any areas of good practice that might be taken up within the home organisation. Such a discussion may well lead to other questions being posed by colleagues that help to expand the learning from the experience.

Support for undertaking learning opportunities in the workplace that require some time out of the work environment will need to be sought from the line manager, and sometimes from others. Ad hoc experiences may be negotiated at any convenient time, but more significant experiences that may impact on the workplace and its staff may be best discussed as part of an appraisal or performance review. You should always have time to plan for a performance review so the more you have thought through your ideas and rationale for the proposal, the better it is likely to be received. Thinking it through should include a clear indication of how the professional development opportunity will benefit the service as well as yourself. Creative ideas for funding may also be relevant to the conversation about the development idea. Longer term workplace learning ideas may include the following:

- A sabbatical or period of unpaid leave, for example, to travel internationally for professional development.
- An opportunity to undertake a secondment within the organisation or elsewhere.
- An opportunity to undertake voluntary work overseas.
- An opportunity to undertake project work – full or part time.
- An opportunity to undertake formal study for an academic award.
- An opportunity to undertake research.

Of course the line manager does not have to agree to any such proposal. However, stressing the benefits for the service may help support the application.

Transforming ourselves

There are clear expectations of health professionals to engage in CPD in order to maintain and develop their competence and to fulfil mandatory CPD requirements. Gonczi (1999) remarked that what constitutes competence in an occupation constantly evolves as new situations are encountered. The more the people engage in work, the more they increase their understanding of both their occupation and their workplace. Additionally, in engaging in activities at work that further develop their knowledge and experience in health and social care provision, health professionals are also taking steps to develop themselves as professional artists. Higgs and Titchen claim that professional practice:

> is a rare blend of people-centred and interactive processes, accountability and profes-
> sional standards, practice wisdom, professional artistry, openness to knowledge growth
> and practice development and engagement in professional journeys towards expertise
> (Higgs & Titchen, 2001, p. 5).

This statement illustrates the multiple demands of professional practice that take place within an environment that is complex and influenced by culture and a high degree of uncertainty. Uncertainty in the workplace can take various forms. Mullavey-O'Byrne and West (2001, p. 55) offer some examples:

- Insufficient funding to adequately maintain services.
- Changing professional roles in the restructured system.
- Increasing demands on practitioners in health care settings.
- Demands and expectations of professional organisations.
- Continual restructuring in some areas, leading to instability.
- Redistribution of resources.
- The virtual disappearance of professionally based allied health departments.
- Changing structures and processes for service delivery.

Yet individual practitioners can use uncertainty to become innovative (Mullavey-O'Byrne & West, 2001). Practitioners can engage with this environment to help transform the lives of people they serve and, through that, to develop their own practice wisdom and also their creative capacity to transform themselves and their world of practice. The practice environment, with all its challenges, ambiguities, uncertainties and complexity, provides the backdrop to the work of the professional who, in his or her world, is striving for competence, proficiency and expertise. Uncertainty and ambiguity in the workplace will continue, so wise practitioners will use that environment to their advantage and demonstrate creativity and innovation in the process of transformation.

Transforming practice

Developing professional practice in the workplace is not just about extending the practitioner' CPD profile, it is a wider professional responsibility. For most practitioners there is a mandate from the relevant regulatory body requiring professionals to engage in CPD and to demonstrate that the CPD has brought about improvement in practice and service delivery to clients. However, developing professional practice can also mean contributing to the transformation of practice. These ideas have, for a long time, been expounded by such learned academics as Ronald Barnett, who argued that all practising professionals had responsibilities that extended beyond those that advanced personal competence to those that advance the profession itself (Barnett, 1994). He went on to remark that confidence of the professional, especially in the light of uncertainty, appeared to be the key to challenging professional practice, which often meant challenging long-held traditions (Barnett, 2000).

Titchen et al. (2001) have also reminded us that professional practitioners face external pressures in the workplace to modify and improve practice in the light of changing circumstances. In order to do this successfully, practitioners ideally need to have developed skills in facilitating change and in using research and evaluation methods effectively to argue their case. Even so, there is no guarantee of success, however well intentioned. Workplaces can be complex and dynamic environments and despite arguments for change to ensure the continued provision of quality services that are relevant and cost effective in a competitive external environment, the long-held traditions may be hard to break. Very often the first challenge of transforming practice has first to be to transform the culture and in particular to develop a learning culture within the organisation. Titchen et al. define a learning culture as:

> the shared vision, meanings, values, beliefs and attitudes held by the organisation and those who work within it, that support learning at work (Titchen et al., 2001, p. 194).

Work on developing a learning culture may take time but is likely to reap rewards especially as the pace of change quickens in the drive to manage competition. There has to be a will to change, for change to be effective, even though it is deemed a professional responsibility. Addressing issues of confidence and any fears of loss may speed the process. However, services cannot stand still and the more the health professionals can develop the skills to advance and transform practice through work-based learning initiatives, the stronger they will be in making their contribution to health and social care.

Organisational culture and communities of learning

Workplace learning focuses on learning that occurs in organisations where the learner is also an employee or a student undertaking a placement. As compared with learning that occurs in an academic environment, the sociocultural aspects of organisational life play a significant part in workplace learning. Political, economic, social and technological issues can impact on the learning experience. These influences serve as a backdrop to work practices and decision-making within the organisation. Learning in the workplace can thus be a more complex affair than learning through tasks, problems or cases presented in an academic setting. However, the workplace can provide both a realistic and rich environment in which to learn. Tennant (2000) proposed that students in particular required a different set of skills for workplace learning reflecting the need to learn from experience. These included the ability to analyse workplace experiences, recognise organisational culture and learn with and from others. Effectively, students needed to become part of the community of learning and contribute accordingly.

Employees will almost certainly find themselves operating within one or more community of practice with its allied responsibility as a community of learning. Wenger (2000) argued that communities of practice form the basis of the social learning system. Through participation in the community the competence of the community is defined. Within a health or social care organisation there are likely to be many communities of practice, some related to individual professions and others related to multi-disciplinary teams that undertake particular functions within the organisation. Members of the community are bound together for a defined common purpose, building their community through mutual engagement in common practices and routines. As a community of practice, the community also becomes a community of learning that promotes its own development by recognising gaps in knowledge, being open to new ideas and opportunities and maintaining a spirit of inquiry. Every individual is thus a contributor drawing on personal experience as a learner to enable the community to enhance, and so redefine, its competence. Abrandt et al. (2004) argued that social interaction within the community about the learning that an individual has experienced not only enhances the learning but also becomes a transformative process for the whole community.

International perspectives on work-based learning

The relevant official regulator of health and social care professionals in different countries of the world sets out the expectations of many of these practitioners with regard to their CPD. Some professions do not have a separate regulatory body and thus still take their guidance from a professional body. This guidance sets out the expectations of practitioners, in particular how they must fulfil any legal requirements as laid down by different countries, states, departments, provinces or other geographical divisions. These measures are primarily intended to ensure public protection. The responsibility lies with individual practitioners to fulfil the correct requirements for the country in which they wish to work. Support from the workplace to promote professional development and fulfil statutory requirements may not ensue. Individuals will thus need to determine their own strategy for improving and updating their practice knowledge to ensure that the public continues to receive the best possible service. However, both national and international collaborations can help meet the needs of professionals in their respective environments. Joint ventures, projects, research, exchange programmes or projects undertaken as visiting practitioners, teachers, scholars or volunteers can provide excellent learning opportunities, in particular, opportunities for comparing and contrasting practice in the different places. New insights into practice can result. Discussions and reflections on conversations may lead to new directions in practice. These learning opportunities all count as professional development.

Some advances have been made in Europe. The NHS European Office is working on policies aimed at promoting the mobility of health professionals across Europe. At the time of writing it is not clear which professions are to be included. However, key areas to be addressed in the proposals include competence to practise and language competence. Recommendations about updating skills can also be anticipated. Work is being undertaken with regulatory bodies to promote better flow of information between countries and other measures to ensure public protection (http://www.nhsemployers. org/EmployabilityPolicyAndPractice/Euro; accessed 22 November 2011).

European lifelong learning strategies have already led to initiatives aimed at 'Tuning' the curricula of the professions for compatibility across Europe. Both social work and occupational therapy curricula have undergone this process and the work has been formally validated by key stakeholders. In relation to Tuning, learning outcomes have now been expressed in terms of the level of competence to be obtained by the learner and recognised at the point of qualification. Tuning provides a benchmark for qualifying courses of the same profession across Europe (University of Deusto & University of Groningen, 2008). All these initiatives are intended to facilitate mobility of staff employed in health and social care environments or seeking learning opportunities in different European countries. The Tuning programme (established to accompany the Bologna Process) lays a foundation of compatibility between qualifying programmes of the same profession. Employability initiatives aim to promote mobility and the uptake of practice opportunities across Europe. Longstanding initiatives that continue to support lifelong learning in Europe include the Erasmus, Leonardo da Vinci and Grundtvig educational programmes. Individuals can apply to these programmes for support for lifelong learning opportunities across Europe.

Other initiatives for supporting the professional development of mid-career professionals in countries beyond Europe include scholarships awarded by the Commonwealth Scholarship Commission. There are various programmes for those from commonwealth countries who wish to visit organisations in the United Kingdom or undertake a short course, and for those from the United Kingdom who wish to visit another country for professional development. These are expenses paid trips of about 3 months' duration to a named host organisation to undertake approved projects of personal/professional interest. The specific criteria are available on the website: cscuk.dfid.gov.uk/apply/professional-fellowships/.

Summary

This chapter has explored ways in which learning in the workplace may be undertaken to aid CPD. Informal experiential learning and more formal academic work are described as possible avenues for learning. It has been shown that there are various ways in which health professionals might engage in learning in the workplace but all are subject to organisational influences that can either help or hinder such learning. Much informal learning has to be initiated by the practitioner. Access to academic courses that either require time off for attendance at university during work time or that are planned as work-based learning modules to be addressed at work may need to be more formally negotiated with a line manager. Many institutions of higher education are now offering academic modules that can be pursued in practice but where the assessments are sent to the university for marking by lecturers. Some formally approved academic modules can be taken online at a time of day that suits the student. Other smaller online modules developed by a university may assist with professional updating but may not attract academic credit. Formal qualifications such as Master's degrees and professional doctorates can also be studied on a part-time basis and use the workplace as a primary learning environment. Learning in the workplace can be transformative in that new knowledge can bring changes that ultimately enhance practice and benefit service users.

References

Abrandt DM, Richardson B & Sjöström B (2004) Professions as communities of practice. In: *Developing Practice Knowledge for Health Professionals* (eds J Higgs, D Fish & R Rothwell), pp. 71–88. Butterworth-Heinemann, Edinburgh.

Barnett R (1994) *The Limits of Competence*. Society for Research into Higher Education and Open University Press, Buckingham.

Barnett R (2000) *Realising the University in an Age of Supercomplexity*. Society for Research into Higher Education and Open University Press, Buckingham.

Billett S (1999) Guided learning at work. In: *Understanding Learning at Work* (eds D Boud & J Garrick), pp. 151–164. Routledge, London.

Boud D & Garrick J (1999) Understandings of workplace learning. In: *Understanding Learning at Work* (eds D Boud & J Garrick), pp. 1–11. Routledge, London.

Boud D, Keogh R & Walker D (1985) Promoting reflection in learning: a model. In: *Reflection: Turning Experience into Learning* (eds D Boud, R Keogh & D Walker), pp. 18–40. Kogan Page, London.

Breen R (2005) Work based learning and the NHSU. In: *Work-based Learning in Health Care: Applications and Innovations* (eds K Rounce & B Workman), pp. 161–170. Kingsham Press, Chichester.

Clarke DJ & Copeland L (2003) Developing nursing practice through work based learning. *Nurse Education in Practice*, **3**, 236–244.

Garrick J (1999) The dominant discourses of learning at work. In: *Understanding Learning at Work* (eds D Boud & J Garrick), pp. 217–231. Routledge, London.

General Social Care Council (2005) *Post-qualifying Framework for Social Work Education and Training*. General Social Care Council, London.

Gonczi A (1999) Competency-based learning: a dubious past – an assured future. In: *Understanding Learning at Work* (eds D Boud & J Garrick), pp. 180–195. Routledge, London.

Higgs J & Titchen A (2001) Framing professional practice: knowing and doing in context. In: *Professional Practice in Health, Education and the Creative Arts* (eds J Higgs & A Titchen), pp. 3–15. Blackwell Science, Oxford.

Jarvis P (2001) The changing educational scene. In: *The Age of Learning: Education and the Knowledge Society* (ed. P Jarvis), pp. 27–38. Kogan Page, London.

Johns C (2002) *Guided Reflection: Advancing Practice*. Blackwell Publishing Ltd., Oxford.

Kember D (2001) Reflections on reflection. In: *Reflective Teaching and Learning in the Health Professions* (eds D Kember et al.), pp. 167–175. Blackwell Science, Oxford.

Kolb D (1984) *Experiential Learning: Experience as a Source of Learning and Development*. Prentice Hall, Englewood Cliffs, NJ.

Lemanski T, Mewis R & Overton T (2011) *A Introduction to Work-based Learning: A Physical Sciences Practice Guide*. The Higher Education Academy, York.

Marsick VJ & Watkins KE (1990) *Informal and Incidental Learning in the Workplace*. Routledge, London.

Morley M (2007) Building reflective practice through preceptorship: the cycles of professional growth. *British Journal of Occupational Therapy*, **70** (1), 1–3.

Mullavey-O'Byrne C & West S (2001) Practising without certainty: providing healthcare in an uncertain world. In: *Professional Practice in Health, Education and the Creative Arts* (eds J Higgs & A Titchen), pp. 49–61. Blackwell Science, Oxford.

Ramage C (2005) It's hard work. In: *Work-based Learning in Health Care: Applications and Innovations* (eds K Rounce & B Workman), pp. 99–111. Kingsham Press, Chichester.

Richardson B, Abrandt Dahlgren M & Higgs J (2004) Practice epistemology: implications for education, practice and research. In: *Developing Practice Knowledge for Health Professionals* (eds J Higgs, B Richardson & M Abrandt Dahlgren), pp. 201–220. Butterworth-Heinemann, Oxford.

Rounce K & Workman B (2005) Introduction to work-based learning in health and social care. In: *Work-based Learning in Health Care: Applications and Innovations* (eds K Rounce & B Workman), pp. 1–11. Kingsham Press, Chichester.

Rounce K, Garlick H, Vernon L & Portwood D (2005) The development of a doctorate in professional studies in health. In: *Work-based Learning in Health Care: Applications and Innovations* (eds K Rounce & B Workman), pp. 145–160. Kingsham Press, Chichester.

Schön D (1983) *The Reflective Practitioner*. Basic Books, New York.

Tennant M (2000) Learning to work, working to learn: theories of situational education. In: *Working Knowledge: The New Vocationalism and Higher Education* (eds C Symes & J McIntyre), pp. 123–134. The Society for Research into Higher Education and Open University Press, Buckingham.

Titchen A, Butler J & Kay R (2001) Transforming practice. In: *Professional Practice in Health, Education and the Creative Arts* (eds J Higgs & A Titchen), pp. 185–198. Blackwell Science, Oxford.

UK Council for Graduate Education (2002) *Professional Doctorates*. UKCGE, Dudley.

University of Deusto & University of Groningen (2008) *Tuning Educational Structures in Europe: Reference Points for the Design and Delivery of Degree Programmes in Occupational Therapy*. Publicaciones de la Universidad de Deusto, Bilbao.

Wenger E (2000) Communities of practice and social learning systems. *Organization,* **7** (2), 225–246.

Chapter 8

Scholarly activity and research for the practitioner

This chapter addresses:

1. reasons for, and ways of, seeking higher academic qualifications to enhance practice;
2. the characteristics of various taught higher degrees;
3. research and independent study as a basis for an academic award.

Introduction

Allied health professionals and social workers gain their qualification to practise in their profession through formal academic learning that leads to a diploma, bachelor's or Master's degree or professional doctorate in the named profession. There are significant variations in the level of the basic academic qualification across the world even within the same profession. The minimum level of qualification may be dictated by either the regulatory or professional body. In some countries, additional profession-specific examinations must be taken and passed after the initial educational qualification is awarded in order to gain a license to practise. Regardless of the level of qualification, most newcomers to a profession are only likely to practise at a basic level of competence during the early part of their career. Professional competence that includes gaining confidence to practise will develop over time and may be dependent on the range of experience gained in the early career stages. Newly qualified practitioners will still need to develop their portfolio of learning in readiness for the continuing professional development (CPD) audit administered by the regulatory body even though they may not be subject to the same level of CPD requirements as their more experienced counterparts in the first year or so of practice. The range of activities undertaken to develop competence is likely to be unique to each individual. Most practitioners are likely to attend practice-related courses in order to gain experience and improve confidence and competence with service users. However, at some stage of a career some practitioners may seek to further their

---

Continuing Professional Development in Health and Social Care: Strategies for Lifelong Learning, Second Edition. Auldeen Alsop.
© 2013 John Wiley & Sons, Ltd. Published 2013 by John Wiley & Sons, Ltd.

academic qualifications and engage in continuing professional education. Roberts (2002) points out that CPD might be a desired effect of continuing professional education, however it cannot be assumed. Both Roberts (2002) and Barnet (1997) note the importance of building critical self-reflection into the educational process to enhance the learning that transpires. It is universities that tend to offer the academic courses, the academic environment and the critical space in which practitioners can engage in dialogue and critical debate with peers about issues that affect them all (Alsop & Lloyd, 2002). These days, the 'environment' of the university extends beyond the physical academic environment into the workplace and to the home environment to meet the different learning needs of students. Courses are thus structured to develop critical reflection in different situations so as to maximise learning.

Reasons for seeking higher qualifications

Many academic programmes delivered by institutions of higher education are offered to assist practitioners to develop and enhance their knowledge base in a chosen area of practice. Understanding the levels of the different awards in higher education is useful so that appropriate choices may be made in the pursuit of academic qualifications. Most people would look to climbing the academic ladder from bachelor's to Master's degree and then to a doctorate. However, there may be very good reasons for gaining another award at the same academic level as the first degree achieved. It is important to make informed choices about the qualification in relation to its value to practice and its potential to support a career or career move. Gaining additional academic qualifications can enable practitioners to do the following:

- Use skills of critical reflection as an aid to learning.
- Develop intellectual skills and academic knowledge for personal gratification and reward.
- Undertake a focused, structured programme of learning with a view to upgrading professional knowledge and skills and maintaining competence to practise.
- Add to existing professional knowledge or skills, for example, by pursuing another recognised professional award such as a diploma in counselling and so provide wider scope for professional practice.
- Supplement the professional award with a recognised management qualification, for example the Diploma in Management Studies (DMS) or Master of Business Administration (MBA) in order to progress a career in management.
- Supplement the professional award with a recognised teaching qualification to enhance skills and to be able to facilitate learning in others. This might open up sessional work with students in the local university.
- Pursue higher level studies in a specialist area that might both enhance practice and intellectual capacity. This might lead to gaining advanced practitioner status or a post in higher education.

- Gain experience, under supervision, of carrying out research in order to be able confidently to seek evidence for best practice or to promote and support research within the service.
- Gain broader-based knowledge and skills or a deeper understanding of practice and organisational issues in order to develop career opportunities or strengthen an application for career progression.

Higher level qualifications may introduce the learner to research techniques, enabling that person to experience research at first hand. The process offers the ability to:

- develop techniques of searching and critically appraising literature;
- critically analyse research papers;
- apply research skills and methods in practice;
- analyse findings and consider their application to practice;
- develop the art of communicating research findings both orally and in writing.

As a minimum, the higher education programme should enable the development of intellectual skills, such as those used in reflection, reasoning, processing information, making judgements, developing arguments, skills in written communication and significant skills in critical appraisal and evaluation. These are skills useful, not just in clinical areas but also in education, management and research. Furthermore, opportunities to identify and discuss espoused theory and theories-in-use should be built into continuing professional education programmes so that the learner can actively engage in processes that explore and test out the practice environment (Roberts, 2002). There is no doubt that undertaking post-graduate study helps an individual to develop confidence as well as personal and professional skills. Those who undertake higher education are generally preparing themselves to be leaders in their profession in one way or another.

Any degree course, at whatever level, offered by a university has been developed and approved as meeting at least the national standards required of a higher education programme. Anyone signing up for a higher degree programme can thus be assured of the quality of education to be received. This makes such a course different from some ad hoc professional courses that are developed for CPD purposes only. That is not to say that such courses have no value, indeed the opposite is almost certainly true as shorter, focused courses dealing with highly specialised practices can be extremely useful in developing the workforce. However, unless previously designed and delivered in association with a university, there is usually no awarding body to confirm the quality of the course. There may be no assessments so the competence of participants taking the course has not necessarily been tested out. Exceptionally, there are some course providers who operate by renown having developed and delivered courses in specialist areas of practice for many years yet have no links to a university. Their own assessment is the test of competence and certificates of attendance or course completion are awarded accordingly. Additionally, some professional associations do offer courses that help develop professional knowledge and skills by drawing on the expertise of those in the field. Experts develop the programme and sometimes review the work of course participants. Some of these may be distance learning or online courses that can be studied at home but will not result in academic credit or qualification. Some work-based specialist programmes may be developed in association with institutions of higher education and formally approved by the university so that professionals gain the formal academic awards on completion of the programme.

Above all, the gain that comes from taking a higher degree programme is the development of advanced levels of critical thinking that help practitioners to feel more confident in themselves and in their work. Most practitioners with a bachelor's degree who are seeking further qualifications would look to undertake a Master's degree some time after gaining their initial professional qualification; a small minority of those holding bachelor's or Master's degrees might apply directly to a doctoral programme. This chapter explores some of the advantages of undertaking scholarly activity for personal reasons as well as for CPD. Firstly, it is worth considering the hierarchy of academic qualifications and the qualities and skills that they help to develop.

Typical higher education qualifications

Table 8.1 sets out a common framework of higher level academic qualifications and identifies some of the awards that are offered by universities in the United Kingdom at the different levels of scholarly activity. Table 8.1 shows awards from Higher National Diploma at academic level 5 to doctoral programmes at academic level 8. Academic levels 7 (Master's level) and 8 (doctoral level) are the ones that most health and social care practitioners will pursue for the purposes of continuing professional education. Table 8.2 shows the knowledge, skills and competence expected of those who achieve a Master's degree or doctorate.

Some specialist programmes are delivered in association with institutions of higher education so that professionals can gain the formal academic award on completion of the programme. An example of this is the UK post-qualifying framework for social work education and training (General Social Care Council, 2005). This framework is said to build on the qualifying degree for social workers and to provide ways in which social workers can maintain and improve knowledge and skills. It takes the view that academic and professional learning should be integrated. Programmes of learning developed as modules and leading to university awards that meet the Council's requirements will be approved but they must be linked to a specific academic level. For specialist and advanced practice the minimum academic level is Master's level. However, this framework is also open to members of other professions, should the modules suit their needs. In this way, inter-professional education is promoted.

The European Qualifications Framework for Lifelong Learning, completed in 2006 (www.ec.europa.eu/education/pub/pdf/general/eqf/leaflet_en.pdf; accessed 25 September 2012) provides a common European reference system for national qualifications that is compatible with the qualifications framework for higher education developed under the Bologna Process, especially for academic levels 5–8. There are eight academic levels in total. Levels 5–8 are used in higher education across Europe.

Table 8.1   Typical awards at academic levels 5–8.

Higher education qualification	Academic level

Doctoral degree
• Degrees based on original research
  ○ Doctor of Philosophy (PhD, DPhil)
• Degrees with taught and research elements
  ○ Doctor of Business Administration (DBA)
  ○ Doctor of Education (EdD)
• Professional doctorates that aim to develop expertise in professional practice
	8

Master's degree
• Longer, research-based Master's degree
  ○ Master of Philosophy (MPhil)
• Master's degrees with taught element and research
  ○ Master of Research (MRes)
  ○ Master of Arts (MA)
  ○ Master of Science (MSc)
• Post-graduate diploma (PgDip): a programme of study normally shorter than a Master's degree
• Post-graduate certificate (PgCert): a programme of study normally shorter than a PgDip
	7
	
	7

• Bachelor's degree with honours: BSc Hons, BA Hons • Bachelor's degree: BSc, BA • Graduate diploma: DipHE • Graduate certificate: Cert HE	6
• Foundation degrees in science or arts: FdSc, FdA • Diploma of higher education: Dip HE • Higher national diploma: HND	5

The European Qualifications Framework indicates expected learning outcomes in terms of knowledge, skills and competence to be achieved at each of the eight reference levels. Table 8.2 shows the knowledge, skills and competence that students are expected to have achieved at levels 7 and 8. These are the two highest levels of academic awards pursued by those practising in health and social care who are undertaking continuing professional education and seeking higher level qualifications. The attributes of levels 1–6 can be found through the website above.

Master's degrees

As well as different levels of qualification there are also different types of qualification at levels 7 and 8 – taught degrees and research degrees. Each makes different demands of students and yields different rewards. Most Master's degrees are taught degrees. These generally comprise taught elements often delivered as modules, each of which has a credit rating and is assessed. Initially, a student aiming for a Master's degree would study for a post-graduate certificate. In the United Kingdom, the post-graduate certificate has a value of 60 Master's (M) level credits. On successful completion

Table 8.2   Knowledge, skills and competence expected of those who pursue Master's degrees or doctorates.

Academic level	Knowledge	Skills	Competence
7 – Master's level	Highly specialised knowledge, some of which is at the forefront of knowledge in a field of work or study as the basis for original thinking and/or research.Critical awareness of knowledge issues in a field and at the interface between different fields.	Specialised problem-solving skills required in research and/or innovation in order to develop new knowledge and procedures and to integrate knowledge from different fields.	Manage and transform work or study contexts that are complex, unpredictable and require new strategic approaches.Take responsibility for contributing to professional knowledge and practice and/or for reviewing the strategic performance of teams.
8 – Doctoral level	Knowledge at the most advanced frontier of a field of work or study and at the interface between fields.	The most advanced and specialised skills and techniques, including synthesis and evaluation required to solve critical problems in research and/or innovation and to extend and redefine existing knowledge or professional practice.	Demonstrate substantial authority, innovation, autonomy, scholarly and professional integrity and sustained commitment to the development of new ideas or processes at the forefront of work or study contexts, including research.

Source: The European Qualifications Framework for Lifelong Learning (2005) © European Union, 1995–2012.

of the relevant modules the student would continue and take further modules to complete a post-graduate diploma, which then replaces the post-graduate certificate. The post-graduate diploma has a total value of 120 M level credits, which include the 60 credits from the post-graduate certificate. When these modules are passed, the student can continue to the final and normally the research phase in order to complete the Master's degree. This often entails undertaking a small-scale research study that has a value of 60 credits, although there are variations to credit values for the research element in some Master's degrees. Therefore, a Master's degree in the United Kingdom comprises modules that total 180 M level credits. Although Master's degrees can be taken and completed through 1 year of full-time study, the three phases of the degree lend themselves to being delivered and completed part time over a 3-year period. Many students of the health professions study part time as this fits best with employment.

Some health professionals lack confidence in their ability to study at Master's level. By signing up initially for a post-graduate certificate, their academic ability is put to the test. Once on the programme, it is frequently realised that the Master's degree is achievable and students pass from year to year quite naturally to complete the full programme. Occasionally, studies are found to be quite testing and incompatible with life circumstances. Some students just complete the first level and walk away with the post-graduate certificate. Sometimes it is possible to complete the Master's degree at a later date. This depends on university regulations. Even if the post-graduate certificate or post-graduate diploma only is awarded, this is still an achievement. This continuing education has undoubtedly brought extended skills that can be used in the workplace and that can be logged for CPD purposes.

Research degrees

The Master of Philosophy (MPhil) is the main research degree at academic level 7. This is not a modular degree but one that requires the student to undertake a significant piece of research under the supervision of a research supervisor. Health professionals wishing to undertake an MPhil are usually required to have completed a suitable course on research methods. Entry to the university is usually by interview where the prospective student presents an idea for research. Once accepted and enrolled at the university, the student, under supervision, prepares a formal research proposal that has to be approved by the university. Depending on the proposed study and consideration of its potential impact on health and social services and service users, formal ethical approval may also be required from the NHS or other relevant authorities. The current procedures for gaining ethics approval must be completed before data can be collected. The supervisor will advise on the up-to-date procedures, which tend to change fairly frequently and are thus not covered here.

It can take 4 or 5 years of part-time study to complete the MPhil degree. It normally requires the student to go through the full research process that involves, in brief:

- undertaking a critical evaluation of relevant literature;
- refining the research question;
- establishing and defending the most appropriate methodology and methods, including as necessary the proposed sample of people to be targeted as participants in the study and ethical issues to be addressed;
- generating data;
- analysing data;
- discussing the consequences of the findings and potential application to practice;
- critiquing the research, identifying any limitations;
- writing the thesis;
- placing the research in the public domain through presentation and/or publication.

When applying to undertake a MPhil degree, the choice of university and supervisor should be given some thought, particularly with regard to the compatibility of the proposed research topic with the research interests of prospective supervisors. It is much easier these days to ascertain information on the research interests of university lecturers through the relevant university website. Publications of lecturers who appear to have similar interests can be looked up and some judgements made about compatibility between the lecturer's research interests and those of the practitioner/would-be student. Some supervisors specialise in particular methodologies and this might also influence the choice of supervisor. It is worth making an informal enquiry to the potential supervisor to ascertain his or her interest in the research topic being proposed for study. In order to pursue specific research interests, some prospective students are willing to travel quite some distance to be supervised by an expert in the field. Significant developments in technology now permit communication for supervision in many different ways, including Skype and e-mail, so distance to a university to undertake study of a specialist nature need no longer be an issue. The MPhil student would normally have to defend their work through a viva voce examination before being awarded the degree, although this varies from university to university.

Transfer to PhD

Some MPhil students may discover that their early findings in the research process are quite significant, unique and worthy of further investigation. It is possible that a minority of students who start out originally wishing to undertake an MPhil are advised by their supervisor that their work is of sufficient intellectual worth and originality, and that transferring to a doctoral programme might be feasible. This is a decision that is not taken lightly as the work will need to extend to a deeper and often more complex level if studying for a doctorate. The decision is generally made after about 2 years studying for the MPhil, although that tends to be flexible. A student does not have to agree to move forward with the transfer and can continue with the MPhil as originally intended. However, in order to transfer to the PhD programme a formal application has to be made within the university and, if successful, a process of transfer is put in place. The student has to defend and critique the work undertaken so far, often as a viva with several experts, and has to propose how the work might continue at doctoral level and at a level of originality expected of doctoral research.

The Doctor of Philosophy (PhD or DPhil) is the main research degree at academic level 8. Applicants wishing to undertake a PhD or DPhil will normally undergo a similar selection process to those applying to take an MPhil. Most doctoral students are initially accepted on to a programme leading to an MPhil with the expectation that at the appropriate time a transfer will be sought on to the PhD programme. Those successful at the transfer stage will continue their studies at doctoral level. Doctoral students are normally allocated two and sometimes three supervisors. Each would bring different expertise, sometimes crossing the boundaries of different disciplines. This ensures a breadth of study and that the student learns to manage different perspectives that are brought to the supervisory process. A viva voce examination of the PhD is common in the United Kingdom. Other countries may refer the work to international expert examiners who will assess the thesis and give their findings with regard to the credibility and quality of the research and its application. The university will then decide on whether the degree should be awarded to the student.

Taught degrees at Master's and doctoral level

Taught higher degrees require students to take a number of modules or courses leading to a Master's degree or professional doctorate. As already described, the post-graduate certificate and post-graduate diploma are staging posts to a taught Master's degree. Applications are made directly to the university offering the programme. The qualifications for continuing professional education and development may normally be studied either part time or full time. Details such as these will be found in the university prospectus. Several universities may offer similar programmes leading to the same or similar qualification. Although it might be convenient to study at a local university, it is worth looking carefully at the curriculum of various universities to see which programme best suits needs or is of most interest.

For both Canada and the United States, the lowest qualifying level for the professions of occupational therapy and physiotherapy is now a taught Master's degree. However, these will be subject to a strict curriculum in order to meet professional standards. Some universities in the United States offer professional doctorates at qualifying level for these professions. Continuing professional education is thus most likely to be at PhD level.

Professional doctorates

Unlike a PhD, which is a research-based degree where a thesis forms the basis of the study, a professional doctorate (DProf) is usually a taught programme that links academic learning with practice in the workplace. According to the Quality Assurance Agency for Higher Education (2011, p. 14) a professional doctorate 'provides an opportunity for individuals to situate professional knowledge developed over time in a theoretical academic framework'. Those who prefer to undertake professional doctorates are normally practice-based professionals who seek to develop fresh insights into their practice and to improve their practice expertise. This is a route to a doctorate commonly chosen by health and social care practitioners who wish to focus on exploring the work that they do in service. The professional doctorate programme normally includes structural elements such as lectures, seminars, workshops and other assessed pieces of work then requires an original piece of research.

It is fair to say that the introduction of professional doctorates has not been without criticism. Traditionally, only a research-based doctorate was deemed to embed the qualities associated with doctoral studies, namely originality, rigorous in-depth study supporting theoretical analysis and evaluation of the research and making a significant contribution to knowledge (Winter et al., 2000). As institutions of higher education developed professional doctorates, criticism emerged from some examiners that professional doctorates could not reach the same level of academic rigour as PhDs and so the doctoral status was in question. The DProf thesis or dissertation submitted for assessment tends to be shorter than a PhD thesis on account of other written work already submitted for assessment earlier in the taught programme that counts towards the academic award. It had been argued that there could be insufficient 'space' in a DProf thesis to develop theoretical arguments to the depth required of a doctorate, and hence academic rigour could be in question.

Those undertaking a PhD might commonly take 4–6 years (part time) exploring, critiquing, challenging and developing theories through their research and in their thesis. A professional doctorate programme, on the other hand, might allocate the first 2 years of part-time study to developing students' critical evaluation and research skills, sometimes through an assessed modular programme. The formal research leading to the production of a thesis or dissertation (the terms used vary from programme to programme) as the final product of the DProf programme is then conducted over the final 2 years, and sometimes longer. The professional doctorate is a structured programme providing an opportunity for a number of students, sometimes from different disciplines, to come together to explore, debate and evaluate research material and so learn to exercise judgement as they progress through the course. The PhD is largely a unique programme of full- or part-time study where an individual is guided by a team of supervisors. The PhD and DProf are different programmes with different outcomes. However, Winter et al. (2000) argue that the quality of the thesis submitted by students on either programme can meet the standards of rigour and originality required of those who are being examined for a doctoral degree.

Advancing a career through research

It has already been noted that some professions now study to Master's level in order to gain the initial qualification to practise in their profession. Esdaile and Roth (2003) cited work done by Warren and Pierson (1994) that claimed that those with Master's degrees felt better prepared to engage in work across a broad spectrum of clinical practice, research, teaching and management activities than those with bachelor's degrees. It certainly seems that those with the higher qualifications have more confidence in their work in different fields of practice and with different levels of responsibility. Esdaile and Roth also reported on the merits of scholarship that is driven first by curiosity and that leads to a process of discovery, otherwise termed 'research'. Integration and application of research in practice follows in order to enhance practice. There is then the responsibility to ensure, through professional education, that new knowledge and practices are disseminated to others. Formal research ensures that steps are taken to bring balance and objectivity to the study. So although many qualities of an advanced practitioner can be developed without undertaking a higher degree, it is the capacity to generate and apply new knowledge to practice through rigorous study and scholarship that creates leaders within a profession.

Practitioners tend to want research that is relevant to practice and can be used in everyday practice (Cusick, 2001). Therefore, choosing research methods that are 'practice-friendly' is critical to the practicalities of researching practice, to the credibility of the research and to the potential application of the research findings in practice. Careful selection of methodology can also maximise chances of the research being completed as there are numerous obstacles to be overcome in practice and environmental challenges to be managed to ensure its completion. Methodology must still be subject to research governance to ensure quality of research (Pettican & Bostock, 2009). Cusick thus advocates for more research-sensitive practitioners who can lead research activity in the workplace and add to the professional body of knowledge and thus the credibility of the profession and its practice effectiveness. Collaborative research with practitioners of the same, or different, professions or with academic colleagues may encourage commitment to the work, but may also bring different expectations that have to be managed sensitively.

Knowing how you learn best

The choice of an academic programme needs to relate to a personal/professional development plan. What are your aims for your career? What professional education and qualifications might serve your career best? What qualifications might be required for the next job you have in mind? As well as personal interest and career aims and expectations, the choice of course should also reflect personal preferences about ways of learning. Figure 8.1 suggests some questions to ask yourself in order to establish your preferred ways of learning. Addressing these questions may help you narrow down your choice of course. For example, if you only have limited time in the day to study and feel that distance learning might suit you better, then the Open University courses might be an option. This choice demands commitment to independent learning and the capacity to study alone. That is not to say that there is no support as Open Universities are renowned for offering many kinds of support, however they do not typically include the kind of regular class support that might usually be available in traditional universities. Most health professionals probably prefer to have contact with other students for support and welcome the opportunity to engage in dialogue. Working with others also provides stimulation and the opportunity to exchange experiences and ideas. This may be important if the student population comes from the same profession. However, working with students from a variety of professions brings exposure to different perspectives that can broaden academic thinking. It is important to have a clear view of what kinds of learning opportunities might suit you best, and which learning arrangements would not suit you. This helps make informed choices, or at least to narrow down the options available that might work. It is important to work through this as quite a few students do not think clearly enough about personal preferences and challenges and then end up having to leave their chosen course because their circumstances make it difficult to continue. This is never good for morale, never mind the financial outlay.

Upgrading a diploma to a degree

Those whose basic qualification is a diploma in higher education may look to universities such as the Open University (www.open-university.co.uk) for courses

Mode of learning
- Do you prefer to learn with others or could you study on your own?
- Could you commit yourself to distance learning at home or would you prefer to have direct contact with others in a classroom?
- Would you need regular, face to face contact with a tutor or could you organise your own learning and seek support as you need it?
- Do you need to work within a well-defined timeframe or do you prefer to learn at your own pace and at a time that suits you?
- Would you prefer to be taught on a course or to learn through your own research or investigation?
- Do you prefer to study full time or part time?
- Do you prefer day time or evening study?
- Do you prefer to take examinations or to be assessed through on-going coursework?
- What are your preferred learning styles (activist, reflector, theorist, pragmatist) and what learning strategies do you prefer? What modes of learning would you reject?
- What access do you have to academic programmes and will there be any practical problems (distance, transport, library access)?
- Will you be able to take study leave to attend a course in work hours or will you have to study in your own time?
- Are you sufficiently conversant with information technology to use this medium for your studies? Do you have access to appropriate IT resources?
- What impact, if any, would undertaking any proposed course have on your personal or family life or significant other for the duration of the course?
- Do you have any other commitments that might limit your choice of educational programme?

Subject matter
- Are you seeking profession-specific, general or inter-professional education?
- Are you looking for course content related to a skill, discipline or client group?
- Are you looking for a course whose content is related to your career aspirations in clinical work, management, education, research or consultancy?

Figure 8.1 Learning preferences

that enable upgrading to a bachelor's degree. The Open University in the United Kingdom offers a variety of degrees, not just bachelor's degrees but also Master's degrees and doctorates. When searching for a distance learning qualification it is also worth remembering that a number of countries now have Open Universities, for example Athabasca University (www.athabascau.ca) in Canada and The Open Universities Australia (OUA; www.open.edu.au) where a number of Australian universities contribute courses so maximising choice. Studying with an Open University means that you study at a time convenient to you. The only exception might be where the course requires you to commit to an online group discussion at a particular time. You would need to check the course details to establish the commitments required.

Returning to learning

The experience of returning to higher education can be daunting for some, but once there, the learning environment can be both stimulating and challenging. Higher education provides 'time out' of the work environment, away from its associated pressures to experience a level of personal and professional development that could never be achieved in-house. Meeting up with people who also want to be challenged can enhance the academic experience. Having the opportunity to debate, question and hear other views can be exciting. The experience allows personal and professional growth as well as the development of intellectual skills. It promotes increased confidence, personal management skills and the ability to think creatively. It allows people to develop their true potential and to see how they might use their enhanced skills in the practice setting.

Returning to learning may also be a route back into practice for those who have taken a break and need to regain skills and update knowledge so that Standards of Proficiency can be met for re-registration with the Health and Care Professions Council (HCPC). There are clear guidelines about procedures and tasks that must be undertaken, but before that, taking an academic course that helps redevelop intellectual skills and knowledge may be helpful especially in developing confidence. Lack of confidence is often the key inhibitor of those wishing to return to practise in their profession. There is a fear that all skills will be out of date and that it will not be possible to learn to practise again in the new context of health and social care delivery, given the time lapse and inevitable changes that have taken place. There are many avenues to redeveloping confidence and taking an additional academic course is just one of them.

The experience of higher education, with its purpose of developing critical beings, can bring about what Barnett (1997) termed 'emancipation' for the individual and is an experience to be savoured. The critically reflective processes that are necessarily integral to higher education prompt change in perceptions and often promote a reconstruction of views of the world. Personal values and goals are likely to be redefined as there is heightened awareness of personal capacity, capability and potential. Sometimes it can be a little demoralising to return to the same working environment on completion of a programme of higher level studies. It is worth having a conversation with a line manager in order to determine how newly found skills and knowledge can be put to use for the benefit of the service.

Experiential learning and independent study

Some practitioners may feel that there are particular issues that they wish to explore in or about practice but Master's courses they have found do not address the issues they have identified. Sometimes the issues may lead to a significant research question that might best be explored through formal research within a higher degree, as already described. At other times there are practice questions to be answered or innovations to be implemented and tested out that could form the basis of a small-scale academic study. Many universities now offer M level modules entitled independent studies (or similar) that allow the student to set their own agenda for study. Independent studies are not research studies where formal methodology has to be proposed, they are investigations around an aspect of practice that might take a variety of forms of experiential learning. Independent studies modules expect the student to set learning outcomes for the investigation they wish to pursue. This may involve a critique of relevant literature and then a series of activities that helps to explore and gain an understanding of the practice issue that has been identified. The learning outcomes of the module would need to match up with the level of knowledge, skills and competence established for level 7 Master's level studies outlined in Table 8.2. These learning outcomes would be agreed with a university tutor who will supervise and then assess the study on its completion. The timeframe for the study would also need to be agreed. Any ethical issues arising would need to be addressed before the study progresses. Normally, an independent study would seek to avoid activities that would otherwise require formal ethics approval as a research study. Often local procedures allow for evaluation and similar activities to be undertaken without formal ethics approval. Any health or social care professional is charged with working ethically anyway so would not conduct him or herself in any way that puts people at risk. The independent study modules are formally approved within a broader academic framework or programme and thus attract academic credit that could be put towards gaining a Master's degree.

Meeting the expectations of different people

The one thing to remember when undertaking a course of study as a practitioner, particularly a programme that leads to an academic award, is that ownership and control of the study lies with the student and university. The course may be self-funded but funding may also come from another source such as an employer; so it can easily, but mistakenly, be perceived that ownership of the project remains with the sponsor. This is not so. There may be an agreement or a commitment to a particular study topic that has benefits for the service, but the way it is approached and the slant that it takes will ultimately be for the student to determine unless, of course, there are factors that mitigate against this. However, agreement about the nature of the study must be reached with the service.

If a project (research project, independent study or work-based programme) is undertaken as part of an academic award then supervision for the project will come from the institution of higher education. The guidance given during the project will be aimed at achieving a successful result for the student, with due regard for ethical and other sensitive issues related to the service. The academic tutor will advise on specific issues that need to be addressed, including any consents required from within the service. This also applies to the final report on the project that is submitted for assessment. The final report remains the property of the university in that it fulfils the requirements of the academic programme. Sometimes managers request sight of the report, but this should normally be denied. The report submitted for assessment will relate to the learning outcomes originally agreed with the tutor. Should a report be required for the service, a modified report that deals specifically with the needs of the service should be prepared and submitted. There may be particular sensitivities that need to be addressed appropriately. In these situations, the two reports serve two different purposes and are prepared for two different audiences.

Accreditation of prior (experiential) learning

There are times when a significant amount of learning may have taken place that may never have been acknowledged in academia. Perhaps very skilled work has been undertaken in practice in another country or in a voluntary or other organisation close to home that has never been assessed. Therefore, there has never been any suggestion about claiming academic credit retrospectively for the learning that has derived from these experiences. The post-qualifying framework for social work education and training (General Social Care Council, 2005) looks to enable social workers, and other professionals as appropriate, to apply to an institution of higher education for recognition of relevant previous experience through portfolio-based modules. Experiential learning that is pre-planned normally falls within a system of learning that can be managed and judged from the start. In contrast, where the work has already taken place, evidence of learning from the experience has to be provided in order to gain academic credit. This is known as accreditation of prior experiential learning (APEL). Evidence of learning can be presented in portfolio form for assessment by university tutors, provided the university has a mechanism and regulations that allow this method of assessment.

The prior experiential learning for which academic credit is being sought must equate to the learning that would have been gained by a student following a matched course of study. In the process of examining the work presented in portfolio form, tutors will consider:

- the evidence of learning presented in the portfolio;
- the relevance of the prior learning to the course of study;
- whether the previous learning is out of date or is still current;
- the academic level of the learning that emerges from the evidence presented.

The prior experiential learning has to be shown to be at an academic level equal to the learning that would normally take place while doing the course. For example, if undertaking Master's level studies, the learning that is demonstrated in the portfolio has to show the features of M level scholarly work. The level at which it is assessed will reflect not just new knowledge but also the evaluation and application of that knowledge in practice. Critical awareness of how that knowledge can be used will be required for M level credit. It is a very time-consuming business to put evidence together and demonstrate that this constitutes learning. The evidence has to be summarised and presented in some logical form. That evidence must show how the learning outcomes are met. It will be important to seek guidance on how best to present the material.

There may be no hard and fast rules about presentation. However, it is worth remembering that those judging the work will have no prior knowledge of it. The work must thus be clearly presented with signposts to the material that is critical to the assessment. There is no need to create a large volume of work; in some ways, the sleeker the better. This will show that critical judgements have been made about what is important to demonstrate learning and what evidence is required. Quality not quantity is best. A clear structure with defined sections and an index will assist the reviewer to locate key features of the portfolio in relation to the learning outcomes. The relevance of the material presented should be indicated and pointers should be given to show how the material links with other sections. Hull and Redfern (1996) made some pertinent points, as summarised below:

- It is learning, not experience, that is being assessed.
- The learning that is being demonstrated should be linked to assessment criteria, that is, the learning outcomes.
- The assessor has to be convinced that learning outcomes have been met.

Summary

This chapter has offered a rationale in support of post-qualification higher level academic studies for those working in health and social care. The chapter has outlined some of the academic opportunities available to health and social care practitioners and consideration has been given to both taught and research-based degrees. The general characteristics of Master's and doctoral degree courses have been explained with reference to national norms. Independent studies as options for academic study have also been mentioned, as have specialist practice courses offered by other providers that have no links with institutions of higher education. The process of gaining credit for prior experiential learning has been explained. In selecting the most appropriate CPD course, it is noted that consideration should be given to preferred ways of learning. The needs of those wishing to return to practice and needing to fulfil the requirements of the relevant regulatory body for registration have also been addressed.

References

Alsop A & Lloyd C (2002) The purpose of post-graduate education. *British Journal of Occupational Therapy*, **65**(5), 245–251.

Barnett R (1997) *Higher Education: A Critical Business*. Society for Research into Higher Education and Open University Press, Buckingham.

Cusick A (2001) The research sensitive practitioner. In: *Professional Practice in Health, Education and the Creative Arts* (eds J Higgs & A Titchen), pp. 125–135. Blackwell Science, Oxford.

Esdaile SA & Roth LM (2003) Creating scholarly practice: integrating and applying scholarship to practice. In: *Becoming an Advanced Healthcare Practitioner* (eds G Brown, SA Esdaile & SE Ryan), pp. 161–188. Butterworth-Heinemann, Edinburgh.

General Social Care Council (2005) *Post-qualifying Framework for Social Work Education and Training*. General Social Care Council, London.

Hull C & Redfern L (1996) *Profiles and Portfolios: A Guide for Nurses and Midwives*. Macmillan, Basingstoke.

Pettican A & Bostock J (2009) UK research governance developments: opportunities for therapy research. *International Journal of Therapy and Rehabilitation*, **16**(5), 289–296.

Quality Assurance Agency for Higher Education (2011) *Doctoral Degree Characteristics*. QAA, Gloucester.

Roberts AEK (2002) Advancing practice through continuing professional education: the case for reflection. *British Journal of Occupational Therapy*, **65**(5), 237–241.

The European Qualifications Framework for Lifelong Learning (2006) *The European Qualifications Framework for Lifelong Learning*. European Commission, Brussels.

Warren SC & Pierson FM (1994) Comparison of characteristics and attitudes of entry-level bachelor's and master's degree students in physical therapy. *Physical Therapy*, **74**, 333–347.

Winter R, Griffiths M & Green K (2000) The 'academic' qualities of practice: what are the criteria for a practice-based PhD? *Studies in Higher Education*, **25**(1), 25–37.

Chapter 9

Learning to write and writing to learn

This chapter addresses:

1. various ways in which writing can contribute to continuing professional development (CPD);
2. ways in which writing skills can be developed and used to communicate with different audiences;
3. partnerships in projects that will help develop confidence to write for publication.

Introduction

Writing is an art that has to be learned and practised. Although it may not immediately be apparent, having the skills needed to record personal plans, write reflectively on events and experiences and present written work effectively in different formats for different audiences will enhance learning in many ways. Professional education provides opportunities for students to set personal goals, reflect on learning experiences and engage in selected forms of scholarly writing. Writing skills should be further practised and developed post-qualification to support learning in and through practice, to help develop practice and therefore to encourage and promote continuing professional development (CPD).

Writing down personal objectives and plans helps focus the mind on future activity. Writing selectively about recent events helps clarify issues that have come to light and new issues that might require further thought and discussion. Reflecting on events helps to draw out and explore the key factors that impacted on the event. Reflections will not necessarily identify all the issues to be resolved. However, writing helps highlight issues that cause dissonance and so prompt debate around issues that should be addressed. Writing reflectively about professional practice is thus concerned with dealing with aspects of service provision that stand out and need to be further understood.

Continuing Professional Development in Health and Social Care: Strategies for Lifelong Learning,
Second Edition. Auldeen Alsop.

Whilst the above forms of writing are personal and not necessarily open to public scrutiny, the ability to write for the attention and interest of others is a more sophisticated skill. Writing for the purpose of providing information, writing to prompt debate and writing to promote change in professional practice not only assists personal professional growth but also assists the development of the profession.

Writing a personal development plan

All health and social care professionals, regardless of the length of time that they have been qualified, should have a personal development plan, as periodically they will be required to verify that they have engaged in a range of CPD activities that ensure that their practice is up to date. The audit undertaken by a regulatory body will require selected professionals to show evidence of having recently undertaken learning activities to update their practice, sometimes in very specific ways. One way of ensuring that professional updating is timely and relevant is to establish a personal development plan. The plan can be recorded electronically within a purposely con-structed framework, such as that provided by PebblePad, or manually in a designated portfolio. The plan should set out clear personal intentions with regard to professional development over a given period of time. As the plans are fulfilled, records of the activities and reflections on the learning from those activities can be added to the portfolio. Revised plans should follow so that learning is continuous in the wider scheme of lifelong learning.

Line managers should take an interest in the development plans of their supervisees as planned professional development activities should align with service needs. Super-vision sessions, performance review meetings or appraisals provide the opportunity to set out objectives for a period of time that will be reviewed in subsequent meetings. The portfolio should show continuous learning using a variety of learning strategies. Larger schemes that support the service, such as projects, will require more detailed plans and timeframes. Project proposals, plans and reports equally provide evidence of CPD. Some individuals may plan to enhance their academic qualifications, whilst others may attempt to write for publication.

Writing learning outcomes

Learning outcomes are useful in particular situations where it is helpful to have a focus on what new learning should be achieved within a given timescale. Some students may be used to preparing learning outcomes that they would expect to achieve by the end of a period of practice or independent learning. These would complement the learning outcomes set by lecturers for coursework but be specific to the particular practice learning environment. Learning outcomes or objectives might be written following an appraisal to serve as a guide for future learning within the service. Any practitioner working on an independent study, whether or not for an academic award (see Chapter 7), would normally set learning outcomes to determine the parameters of the study. Learning outcomes provide clear statements against which evidence of achievement can be matched in order to determine whether the outcomes have been met.

Setting the learning outcomes to be achieved often just means completing a statement, for example:

By my next appraisal I will . . . (e.g.) . . .
. . . critically review at least two recent (within the last 2 years) research-based articles on the management of X condition.
For this independent study I will . . .
. . . critically examine the care management notes of eight clients diagnosed with dementia within the last 6 months to determine the similarities and differences between their perceived social care needs.

In the case of experiential learning, the learning outcomes will be determined through retrospective reflection and critical analysis of what occurred and what has been learned, for example:

As a result of this learning experience I can now . . .
. . . critically differentiate between the roles and functions of members of the care management team.

Case studies

Students often have to present case studies as a means of developing and demonstrating their learning, particularly from practice. However, unusual cases that have challenged more experienced practitioners can equally be used as incidents for learning and for demonstrating CPD at any stage of a career. Cases that have required more thought, more research, more consultation, discussion, professional reasoning and decision-making are those that are worthy of recording as a learning incident. Clearly, anonymity is required if the case is added to the professional portfolio. It is important to document the reasons for perceiving the case to have special value for learning. Any research and reading that has been undertaken in order to better understand the case should be highlighted. Documenting the service user's story, any diagnosis and key factors that make the case different, and options considered in the case management process may also be recorded. The intervention plan, reasons for decisions taken and procedures that went well, those that were discounted or did not work could also be useful for the record. A final review of the learning that has occurred should be added to the case study for the purpose of CPD.

Project proposals

Health and social care professionals from time to time may have the opportunity to undertake a project on behalf of their employing organisation. Projects can take many forms and be triggered in many ways. For example, a project might test proposed changes within the organisation related to working practices or an idea that might improve practice. The project might be exploratory or a pilot for a larger programme of work.

A project is a defined set of coordinated activities carried out in an organised way with an identified start and end point and that aims to achieve specific results within a set budget and other defined parameters. Therefore, a project proposal will address the key elements outlined in the definition. The proposal might also address the following:

- The rationale for the project and any business justification.
- The aim of the project and projected benefits.
- Scope/parameters of the project (what it will and will not include).
- Any identified or potential risks or other constraints.
- Who will lead the project and to whom that person will report.
- The timeframe for each activity and the person responsible for its completion.
- The resources required for the project (physical, financial and human resources and skills).
- The outcomes to be delivered, for example, project interim/final reports.
- Criteria for the success of the project.

On completion of the project, a report should be prepared to address most of the issues above. The report could either be a short executive summary or a full report of the project (or both) as agreed. The report would be an account of the project focusing on its purpose and outcomes, with any future recommendations identified. The report would be largely factual and service benefits deriving from the project would be highlighted. Sometimes different reports are produced for different audiences. Each would only contain information relevant to the specific audience. Any project report might be cited as evidence of CPD especially if it relates to potential benefits for service users. A separate portfolio entry should refer to the project and the report but should offer a reflective account of the process of undertaking the project and consider the specific personal learning that has derived from it.

Writing reflectively

Reflection is essentially a sense-making process undertaken to discover new connections or conclusions that might guide future practice (Savin-Baden, 2008). Continually reflecting in, on and about practice serves to develop expert practice and helps to shape a future profession through the changes that are prompted and the discarding of outdated practices (Abrandt Dahlgren et al., 2004). The process of reflecting on situations alone or through dialogue with others can lead to new insights but new thoughts that lead to new positions or stances can also develop through the process of writing.

Reflective journals

Some practitioners, especially those new to practice, choose to keep a journal of reflections on selected occurrences that have led to new learning. These events may just be short, but meaningful, conversations with others, opportunities to watch others perform a new procedure in practice or a chance to examine and discuss a new piece of equipment for use in practice. In the journal, it is first useful to describe what happened, analyse and identify key features that warrant further thought or action, note any gains from the experience such as application potential or follow-up plans, thus making each event a learning experience. Essentially, the journal can contain a series of notes about new experiences that can affect practice. Keeping a journal not only ensures that new learning is recorded, but also if personal reflections are added the journal can help promote a better understanding of practice. These journals need not exclusively depend on the written word. Some journalists work in pictures, photographs, drawings or sketches or other creative media, or a mixture of several media that capture new experiences. Reflective comments, however short, can bring these artefacts to life in relation to relevance to practice. Technology now allows for journal entries to be made in different modes including in e-journals if desired. Journal entries may be recorded electronically or handwritten in a diary or notebook designated for the purpose. They are suitable records of CPD and, where relevant, can be submitted for the CPD audit of the regulatory body.

Reflections on learning events

Learning can occur in many different ways and from many different experiences. This section deals specifically with learning from planned events such as attending conferences, exhibitions, meetings or visits. The reason for planning to attend such an event normally stems from wanting to update or develop practice knowledge in one way or another. In order to maximise learning from the event some key objectives should first be formulated. This means that time spent at the event can be focused on achieving specific goals and serve as time well spent. Regardless of additional benefits deriving from attendance, at least the objectives for going will be fulfilled. Therefore, writing reflections on the event should be concerned with two observations. Firstly, reflections on the extent to which objectives were met should be noted together with the key learning that resulted from attending to the objectives. Secondly, any further reflections should address additional features of the programme that prompted unexpected learning. It should be possible to list the learning outcomes as an entry for a portfolio and to consider how that learning might subsequently be used in practice. What benefits might derive from the experience for the service and its users? This is key for organisational effectiveness and to justify time spent on attendance. It is difficult enough to take time out of service delivery for learning purposes, given pressures on the service. Evidence of planning for and reflecting on the event will demonstrate that time out of the service was justified. If attending a conference for the purpose of presenting a paper or poster, there is additional material to record. Either presentation will almost certainly have required some research and some time to prepare. It provides additional evidence of learning for a portfolio. Journal entries may form the basis of feedback to others who were not able to attend the event. Many organisers of learning events now issue either a certificate of attendance or a certificate of participation (as appropriate) at the end of the event. This provides evidence of CPD for a portfolio.

Writing in narrative form is part of a reflective, self-conscious and interventionary process where abstract thought is required to determine new interpretations and emerging issues (Freshwater, 2002). Without the reflective component there would only be a story; without the writing, the account may be incomplete. The written account should capture the essence of events; the reflections should address ambiguities and ultimately initiate transformation in practice.

Critical incidents

Critical incidents have been variously defined. Tripp (1993) suggested that the term referred to some event or situation that marked a significant turning point in time. Gould and Masters (2004) considered them to be specific events from practice that challenged understanding or behaviour. Critical incidents tended to be those memorable events that have an emotional impact and eventually trigger change in practice. To record critical incidents, first a factual account of the incident is written down, including the events that led up to the incident. Note should be made of both the immediate and wider context of the incident as these may have a bearing on what happened, and its consequences. Then the incident should be analysed and the consequences of any actions taken should be noted. Careful analysis of an incident may reveal the factors that led to a particularly successful outcome. Equally, an analysis may reveal aspects that led to unwarranted results. The analysis of the incident can lead to new insights that will inform future decision-making. Often the incident can become invested with new meaning and result in some transformation of both understanding and practice. Critical incidents may indicate the need for a case audit to aid learning and improve practice. A case audit assesses what happened in practice against any pre-set quality standards or expectations. Cases that have been particularly difficult to manage or those that have been particularly successful are those that are best analysed to see what lessons can be learned. Improved understanding of the issues should help practitioners to develop 'the best practice' to which all professionals should aspire.

Being critical

Barnett (1997) asserted that the professional world is a multiple world full of alternative possibilities of strategy, action and communication. But in order to perceive alternatives, the individual has to learn to be a critical thinker capable of generating new ideas. Becoming a 'critical being' involves developing critical thought, critical action and critical self-reflection. Through critical self-reflection individuals develop themselves and through critical thinking they develop confidence in forming an opinion. The insight gained through critical practice and through thinking critically about practice allows individuals to develop more efficient strategies for managing the things they have to do. Critical awareness and the learning that derives from it can be developed in a number of ways, all of which can be classified as CPD.

Writing critically

Being critical in reading, in verbal discussion or in writing does not imply criticism. Being critical is concerned with making informed comment and judgements about the topic under review after evaluating the evidence. Other views may be opened up for consideration and possible discussion, and alternative ways of viewing a situation may potentially be put forward. A critique should aim to improve understanding of the issues or at least broaden the perspectives on them whereby other judgements may be made. When critiquing the observations of others, different positions may be adopted. For example, Taylor (1989) proposed the following positions:

- Agreeing with, acceding to, defending or confirming a point.
- Proposing a new point of view.
- Conceding that an existing point of view has merits but could be better qualified.
- Reformulating and providing a new version for a point of view.
- Dismissing a point on account of its irrelevance or inadequacy.
- Rejecting, rebutting or refuting an argument on reasoned grounds.
- Reconciling two positions that may seem at variance or retracting a previous position based on new evidence or argument.

(Taylor, 1989, p. 67, cited in Blaxter et al., 1996, p. 217)

Writing a critical review of topic-specific material found through a literature search, for example, may either help to clarify arguments and establish justification for existing practice, or help to form reasoned proposals for developing new practice. A critical review could offer an historical account of the topic under review and highlight the changes over time as supported by the relevant evidence of the day. New evidence from any recent research may well shed new light on practices that have been 'custom-and-practice' for some time. A critical review would critique the new proposition and the evidence supporting it and would highlight the differences between the various positions. Reviews that explore what others working in a similar field of practice are doing can help bring new knowledge into focus and improve practice effectiveness for service users. Undertaking a critical review of a single article is a good way to start. A more challenging activity would be to undertake a review of a selection of literature on a particular topic relevant to practice and add that to a professional portfolio. The intention is to assess whether practice in a particular area is still current or whether new research has highlighted the need to change practice in any way. Professional journals may have examples of literature reviews as models that can inform newcomers to this form of critical writing. Writing an account of a research project would include a short section on the literature consulted.

Personal challenge

Writing things down can take courage and may not be everyone's preferred mode of communication. Savin-Baden (2008) suggested that sometimes at the heart of writing there could be an element of personal risk particularly as it was necessary often to challenge oneself, adopt a particular stance or position and set out a personal opinion for others to consider and possibly challenge. By their nature, personal reflections are intended to raise issues that have not been satisfactorily resolved. Setting out a reflective position can help open up avenues for a resolution. Personal journal entries will not normally be subject to such challenge. However, it may still be difficult to express personal feelings, concerns and other observations in a journal as writing is perceived to have permanence. Journals are personal; they have no external readership and subsequent entries can supersede and contradict previously recorded thoughts and opinions without consequences. However, those who seek to write for publication may experience challenges from external sources as their work is intended for the public domain.

Writing styles

Every writer will need to find his or her own style, whether for writing in a personal log or for writing for others. Reading articles from different journals, reading dissertations, theses and other reports or participating in a journal club exposes readers to different writing styles. Reading others' work also helps to develop critical skills and the ability to evaluate others' written contributions. Equally, participating in a writing group will provide opportunities for practising the art of expressing thoughts on paper for a particular audience. Writing is a skill and, as with other skills, it improves with practice. Experimenting with different styles of writing will help develop a personal style that is comfortable and that can be used as a style of choice in different situations. However, sometimes it is necessary to conform to a given writing style if writing for a particular journal or audience. The purpose of the work and the audience or readership will dictate the level of formality required of the writing. Writing a personal log or diary can be liberating as it allows complete freedom of writing style as well as content. Writing notes, messages or directions on which others might act demands clarity of the written word. Writing a conversation piece or an opinion piece permits expressions of opinion backed by argument for others to consider and perhaps critique from their own perspective. Writing a scholarly article for a journal has to conform to the author's guide set out by editors of the journal selected for publication of the article, but will almost certainly be a formal piece of writing. Writing a research article normally means following the common conventions of presenting the research process and its findings. Critical analysis and evaluation of others' written work and personal reflections on contributions to academic studies are integral parts of a research report, written dissertation or thesis and are prepared for a selective audience.

Writing is an emotive task that can be pleasurable but equally can be frustrating and even cause distress. Writer's block, as it is sometimes called, is not uncommon, but as Savin-Baden (2008) points out, the blockage may be a form of disjunction characterised by confusion and frustration and sometimes by a loss of sense of self. However, blockages tend to be challenges that have to be managed and resolved, such as lack of ideas, lack of clarity, noise or unwanted interruptions. Lack of confidence can hinder many a potential writer. For example, submission of an article for publication in a refereed journal will be subject to feedback from selected reviewers prior to publication. The intention is for the feedback to be constructive and assist the writer to improve the submission and its relevance to the readership. Much hard work will already have gone into the preparation of the submission so it can be devastating to receive a poorly constructed review that is critical rather than constructive in its tone. The criticism has to be put to one side in order to move forward and work towards improving the piece for publication.

Writing is also a lonely occupation. But for those who persevere, writing, whether for personal reflection or public information, can also be enjoyable, can bring greater clarity to personal thinking and changes in ways of acting and can ultimately bring considerable personal pride and satisfaction at the achievement of seeing work in print.

Developing writer identity

Whilst Barnett (1994) considered it essential for professionals constantly to challenge their practice and develop new knowledge and practice, Savin-Baden (2008) advocated that a further responsibility was to be able to place the new knowledge in the public domain in forms of academic writing. She offered some thoughts about writer identity in that it requires the following:

- Taking a stance towards what is read.
- Discovering and using a writing voice.
- Finding flow.
- Being prepared to take risks with ways of writing and presenting findings.
- Understanding the circumstances when writing most easily takes place.
- An appreciation of the importance of different writing strategies.
- Recognising that writing is a constant challenge to identity and is therefore necessarily troublesome.
- Understanding that multi-modal writing is complex (Savin-Baden 2008, p. 44).

Writer identity implies having the confidence to share personal opinion or a personal interpretation of the work of others, with others, in a public way. Responses may indicate differences of opinion but this is how variations and refinements of practice eventually occur.

Writing for the public

Confidence in writing ability, as described above, is necessary if writing for a wider audience. Most activities involving writing so far described lead to products for personal use and as a possible addition to a portfolio. More challenging projects include the preparation of information leaflets for the public, and practice-based reports, book reviews, literature reviews and other articles for publication in a professional journal. The preparation of research projects, including dissertations and theses for academic awards, can also be counted as more challenging initiatives. However, for these reports academic supervisors will offer guidance and advice. When it comes to writing for publication, most novice writers pair up with more experienced writers in the first instance. For example, acting as a second or third author for an article or a book chapter provides the opportunity to make a contribution to the work and learn the process of submitting the written piece for publication. There will be mutual support in the research and writing process and there will be opportunity to give and receive constructive comment on the piece as a whole prior to its submission. Alternatively, the assistance of a mentor or critical friend who has previously published and thus knows the process can be extremely helpful. A critical friend can comment on a draft of the work prior to submission for publication and help build confidence in writing skills. Academic supervisors will happily guide their students through the publication process and team up with them to promote the publication of an article on issues that have arisen from the research process. The editor of the chosen journal for publication will often advise on submissions, so it is worth making contact with him or her. So help is at hand and novice writers should not be afraid of seeking support in the early stages of publication.

Information leaflets

Health and social care professionals from time to time are called upon to develop an information leaflet for service users. The information leaflet could reflect any aspect of practice. It might describe a new technique or piece of equipment, for example, and give guidance on its use. However, it is essential that the information is clear, concise, accurate and complete. It must be readily understood by those for whom it is intended. It should also indicate where further assistance may be obtained. The compilation of a leaflet may have required research on the topic and on those who might use it and this should be indicated. The research undertaken, the process of compiling the leaflet and the end result can be used as evidence of CPD.

Book reviews

Professionals who have specialist knowledge and experience may be invited to read and review a new book coming on to the market. Preparing a book review for an editor requires critical reading skills and an ability to present a concise, balanced appraisal of the published material, normally within a word limit specified by the editor. The topic of the review is likely to be of interest to the reviewer and as such it presents an opportunity personally to update, broaden or deepen knowledge of the subject. The review will offer an overview of the book with comment about its content and quality and ways in which it might serve as a resource for practitioners. Any particular merits of the book can be indicated together with any significant shortcoming, if applicable. Reviewing books can be a very rewarding activity, providing an opportunity to assess the practice methods and opinions of others with similar interests. The review could become the first publishing experience. It can help build the confidence to submit other, more personal, pieces of work for publication. Writing for publication demands the ability to organise material, make constructive observations, formulate cohesive arguments and manage a discussion in a cohesive way. Writing books requires similar skills and the ability to work with large quantities of material in an organised way. It also requires the tenacity to complete the task! All practice-led publications may count as CPD activity.

Literature reviews

A literature review is a summary and critical evaluation of a selected range of existing literature dealing with knowledge and understanding in a given field. The review provides insights into previous work and often sets the context for new work. Literature reviews can be useful for updating knowledge about a given area of practice and can provide the opportunity to explore what other people are doing in the same field of work. Literature reviews may start off being undertaken as a matter of personal interest on a topic related to practice. Information generated by a review may offer opportunities to liaise with authors (nationally and internationally) about their work and thus to enhance a working knowledge of practice.

A critical review of related literature may be the end product that informs future practice. However, a literature review may also serve as a precursor to a more formal piece of research. It can help determine what other researchers have done in the field and indicate gaps in knowledge of the topic that might help formulate a question for future research. Sometimes the review may be a piece of work commissioned by another person or group of people as part of a wider project. The work involved first requires the parameters to be set for the topic under consideration and the breadth of the search. A systematic search of the literature is then undertaken using specifically designed electronic databases. Sometimes this is supplemented by a hand search of material that selected databases would not bring up. Librarians and staff in learning resource centres are experts in sourcing literature relevant to a given topic and are normally happy to guide and advise in search techniques.

Scholarly work

Scholarly work might include formal reviews of literature, and articles, chapters and books written for publication, especially if underpinned by research. Scholarly work will also include research reports and work presented in a thesis or dissertation that is being prepared for academic examination. Guidance is readily available on how to present this type of work. Authors' guides are available to those who write articles, chapters and books for publication. University guidelines are available to those who are preparing work for examination. Libraries, especially university libraries, will contain many examples of scholarly work, both published and unpublished. Consulting relevant work and examining the style of writing and presentation in various pieces of work will best help those who are in the process of producing similar work themselves.

Creative writing

Creative writing is a very different activity to the forms of writing previously discussed. It is included here as another form of learning but one that has no rules and, unless otherwise intended, no readership other than the author. Creative writing is a very personal activity that can become a learning activity often with an added therapeutic value. It can counter the stresses and strains of scholarly writing and other formal work through the production of written material where no judgement is offered on what is recorded. Bolton promotes creative writing as a simple, quiet, private, focused activity for personal reflection. Some people keep a personal journal for reflections on daily activities. Sometimes the additions to a journal are in the form of creative writing that can help self-understanding, alleviate distress and improve well-being (Bolton, 2011). Johnson (2001, p. 66) perceived that a journal was where 'memory and meaning finally meet'. Alsop (2002, p. 197) noted that 'a journal is a place where questions are raised, where feelings and emotions are expressed and perhaps where resolutions are proposed for the future'.

This personal form of writing can be read, re-read, reflected upon, developed, redrafted and later shared with others, if required. Writing in this way offers the opportunity to view topics and scenarios from different perspectives. It helps with the exploration of areas that are unknown and with the discovery of insights and personal feelings into selected life events. The creativity embedded in creative writing encourages learning. It can affect both the self- and worldview because it is attained through experience, exploration and expression rather than instruction (Bolton, 2011, p. 17). Creative writing is about freedom of expression but with the benefit of potentially developing new wisdom. After careful thought and consideration, some of the 'gems' (Alsop, 2002) that have been recorded in a personal journal that have prompted new ways of thinking, doing and advancing practice may find themselves in a portfolio or be considered worthy of wider publication.

Summary

This chapter has considered various ways in which developing and using writing skills can contribute to personal learning and professional development. Preparing a personal development plan and making entries in a personal portfolio are activities that can help focus the mind towards achieving career goals. Ways of writing reflectively and creatively help develop new insights into practice and innovative ways of advancing practice. Writing formally is often necessary when undertaking an academic programme leading to a higher degree. The ability to write clear learning outcomes is a skill to be acquired for focusing and guiding academic work to maximise chances of success. Engaging in academic studies also requires the ability to write critically and make judgements supported by evidence. Clearly presented case studies that evidence new learning can provide records of unique experiences with service users and also count as CPD. Ways of presenting written work must be selected as appropriate for the purpose of the work, so developing a range of writing styles is important. Writing effectively is not always an easy skill to learn and apply in different situations.

Feedback from colleagues can be useful and should encourage the development of appropriate writing styles. Writing for publication to disseminate new knowledge is a professional responsibility but requires the ability to present information clearly and concisely in accordance with authors' guides.

References

Abrandt Dahlgren M, Richardson B & Kalman H (2004) Redefining the reflective practitioner. In: *Developing Practice Knowledge for Health Professionals* (eds J Higgs, B Richardson & M Abrandt Dahlgren), pp. 15–33. Butterworth-Heinemann, Edinburgh.

Alsop A (2002) Diamonds of the dustheap. Editorial. *British Journal of Occupational Therapy*, **65** (5), 197.

Barnett R (1994) *The Limits of Competence: Knowledge, Higher Education and Society*. The Society for Research into Higher Education and Open University Press, Buckingham.

Barnett R (1997) *Higher Education: A Critical Business*. The Society for Research into Higher Education and Open University Press, Buckingham.

Bolton G (2011) *Write Yourself*. Jessica Kingsley, London.

Freshwater D (2002) Guided reflection in the context of post-modern practice. In: *Guided Reflection: Advancing Practice* (ed. C Johns), pp. 225–238. Blackwell Science, Oxford.

Gould B & Masters H (2004) Learning to make sense: the use of critical incident analysis in facilitated reflective groups of mental health student nurses. *Learning in Health and Social Care*, **3** (2), 53–63.

Johnson A (2001) *Leaving a Trace: The Art of Transforming Life Into Stories*. Little Brown and Company, Boston, MA.

Savin-Baden M (2008) *Learning Spaces*. The Society for research into Higher Education and Open University Press, Maidenhead.

Taylor G (1989) *The Student's Writing Guide for the Arts and Social Sciences*. Cambridge University Press, Cambridge. Cited in: Blaxter L, Hughes C & Tight M (eds) (1996) How to Research. Open University Press, Buckingham.

Tripp D (1993) *Critical Incidents in Teaching*. Routledge, London.

Chapter 10

Career development

This chapter addresses:

1. careers and the rationale for career development;
2. ways of advancing in a career;
3. networks for aiding professional development and avoiding professional isolation.

Introduction

Earlier chapters have introduced the concept of continuing professional development (CPD) as a necessity, both for meeting the requirements of the regulatory body for professional updating and public protection and for keeping abreast of changes in the external environment with regard to employment opportunities. It has been stressed that jobs are no longer for life, that the economic climate creates uncertainty in the job market, that the pace of change has quickened leaving some employees under threat of losing their job and that there can no longer be complacency around job and career prospects. Even in large organisations offering fundamental services in health and social care and employing well-qualified practitioners to meet the ever-increasing needs of service users, there is still uncertainty for the long term. New technology, new government policy and financial constraints can all bring about change that embraces threats as well as opportunities. Therefore, it can be argued that each individual needs a strategy for personal development beyond the minimum expectations of CPD so as to be able to maintain a career and a lifestyle of choice. This chapter explores a more structured approach to CPD advocating the broadening of skills and enhancement of practice in an attempt, not only to promote career development, but also to support some form of job security and satisfaction.

Continuing Professional Development in Health and Social Care: Strategies for Lifelong Learning,
Second Edition. Auldeen Alsop.
© 2013 John Wiley & Sons, Ltd. Published 2013 by John Wiley & Sons, Ltd.

What is a career?

As noted in Chapter 1, Douglas Hall has been one of the key theorists in terms of 'career' and his definitions of career have changed over time, influenced by different theoretical perspectives and environmental factors. An early definition centred on the notions of 'time' and a linear process of work-related activity. In the early days, Hall, with colleagues, defined 'career' as 'an evolving sequence of a person's work experiences over time' (Arthur et al., 1989, p. 8). Later this was modified to a more complex 'working' definition that took account of rather more perspectives, as follows:

> The career is the individually perceived sequence of attitudes and behaviours associated with work-related experiences and activities over the span of the person's life' (Hall, 2002, p. 12).

As Hall points out, this definition focuses more on the subjective career experience of the individual, the way in which the person constructs or enacts the career. This reflects the sign of the times that no longer is a career deemed a continuous set of employment experiences in one organisation. Rather, the term career denotes work and work-related experiences that have been selected by the individual based on a combination of external influences and personal choice guided by attitudes and motivation. Hall (2002) accounted for a career as a process, rejecting the more constraining views of career as a profession or even career as advancement. Work activities that are paid or unpaid can be acknowledged within a career.

According to Woodd (2000), Herriot (1992) had already put forward similar notions of a subjective approach to career that recognised personal beliefs, values, expectations and aspirations. Additionally, environmental factors could potentially impact on choice. Commonly, people react in one of three different ways to external factors: (1) passively, (2) reactively or (3) actively. Individuals can either take control of their future or be swept along by events. These observations point to choices that have to be made. But choice also involves consideration of life plans, career plans and career opportunities, and there may be conflicts between the demands of a personal life situation and personal career aspiration. A personal view of what constitutes success has also to be considered as this will impact on any career decision made. Some theories hold that individuals seek congruence between personality and environment. An environment is sought that offers the individual an opportunity to flourish and succeed. However, personal needs change over time and career decisions tend to depend on the stage of career, the changing influences of family and considerations such as the relative importance of lifestyle, security, pensions and job location. At some stages of a career there may need to be a trade-off between stability and security for future employability, so risks present themselves from time to time. Context remains important but, over time, personal circumstances, values and aspirations change. Career decisions may reflect current circumstances more than longer term aspirations.

Work is valued for many different reasons. Many people seek the opportunity to be creative at work, to use problem-solving skills and deal with challenges, to work autonomously and contribute something of value to the employing organisation (Alsop, 1992). Opportunities at work to fulfil these needs help maintain interest in the work. They help forge the 'psychological contract' between employer and employee and strengthen the natural tie that binds the relationship. It reduces the need to consider change of employment (Whymark & Ellis, 1999) for as long as the opportunities exist and work remains fulfilling. Working within a group and having a connection with others can also be important as is the ability to progress within the organisation, to acquire new skills and develop existing skills to a higher level. Job security is valued and opportunities for advancing within the organisation are welcomed (Yarnall, 1998). Those elements of the work situation act as 'career anchors' (Schein, 1978) to the organisation, yet in times of uncertainty in the employment market these benefits may not be guaranteed. Individuals have constantly to be aware of external influences on organisational structures and take steps themselves to develop assets that are required in a changing world. Challenges in systems of health care require professionals to draw on a rich array of knowledge and skills in order to work in complex systems and environments (Higgs et al., 2004a). Therefore, novice practitioners must learn quickly to survive in such environments and make a valid contribution to the service. Professionals must learn to manage uncertainty in difficult situations in everyday practice. Changing jobs brings its own challenges even where there are perceived rewards. Where there are no family ties, mobility in employment may be possible in order to retain those aspects of work that offer rewards and personal fulfilment. Changing jobs to fulfil personal dreams may be more difficult where there are other family members to consider. So compromises may have to be made. Nevertheless, the aim is to be constantly vigilant in the work environment and to take steps towards developing skills and talents so as to maximise potential to take up opportunities that are presented, in essence to survive and thrive.

Career development

It has been noted above that the notion of 'career' has been changing over time so that there is now much more uncertainty about ways in which any career is going to pan out. However, this does not mean that careers cannot be planned, it just means that the planning may have to take account of that uncertainty. The planning has to be more flexible so that opportunities can be taken up as they arise. For example, career opportunities may lead to a sideways move within an organisation rather than a promotion. Nevertheless that move may lead to skill enhancement and to opportunities for developing and using talents in different ways. Being prepared to move in any direction shows flexibility in practice. Work-related opportunities become CPD opportunities and thus can be viewed as an investment in time and energy so that talents can be broadened and strengthened in readiness for another move.

A planned and structured approach to career development is important. However, at the same time it is necessary to keep an eye on any significant environmental changes that could impact on organisations and influence decisions. Awareness of context helps maintain a competitive advantage over others. Sometimes it is worth considering how an organisation is working and the extent to which it is moving in different directions. Professional development opportunities may arise from reorganisation or shifts in business planning. At other times it may be necessary to plan for career changes beyond those that might be available within the current employing organisation. These may make more personal demands, but if the current organisation fails to support CPD initiatives then alternative employment may offer better conditions.

Individuals do want to succeed at work and achieve things for themselves. Where there are specific plans, these serve as a guide to activities that lead to attainment. As goals are reached, these act as markers and achievements in the overall plan. Career commitment is defined as 'the extent to which someone identifies with and values his or her profession or vocation and the amount of time and effort spent acquiring relevant knowledge' (Goulet & Singh, 2002, p. 75). It has to be noted here that this definition favours a commitment to a profession rather than a commitment to an organisation. The latter is more readily explained through the term psychological contract. Research reported by Goulet and Singh (2002) suggested that employees would be more committed to their career if their current job were in line with career aspirations but also suggested that an employee is unlikely to continue to display career commitment and loyalty as jobs became less secure. These observations link back to comments in Chapter 1 about 'protean careers' where the focus is more on personal self-development than on a commitment to a job, and increased likelihood of job mobility in order to retain employment.

Advancing in a career

In order to advance a career, an individual has to be proactive. There can be no reliance on other people for assistance, although some mentors (friends, relatives, line managers or others) may be supportive and offer guidance about how to move forward. Each individual also has to have some idea of what will provide satisfaction in a career and take responsibility for planning to ensure that it is achieved. Some people like the security of a job and will take steps to become an expert in a field of practice without seeking new employment or roles. Others will develop knowledge and experience and so broaden their skills with sideways moves, taking on additional responsibility or roles, furthering their knowledge through teaching experience or undertaking research. It is a responsibility of all professionals to generate new knowledge and so to develop the knowledge of their profession for professional growth (Barnett, 1997; Higgs, 2003). Practitioners should thus take responsibility at least for suggesting areas of research. The ability to do this derives from a capacity to critically evaluate personal performance as a means of becoming aware of emerging issues in practice (Higgs et al., 2004a). Research helps consolidate and extend knowledge and develop skills of critical thinking. Advancement in a career is aided by the development of what Higgs et al. (2004b) term professional artistry, which they portray as a creative, advanced way of knowing; the epitome of professional judgement and reasoning ability. They concur with Beeston and Higgs (2001) that professional artistry is exhibited by individuals who possess both artistic and expert qualities that have been developed through extensive and reflective individual knowledge and experience. Many, often invisible, factors are thought to underpin the decisions of practitioners using professional artistry, for example, values, beliefs, attitudes, expectations and feelings as well as knowledge (Fish, 1998). The practice of reflection and critical thinking will help hone the skill of bringing multiple factors into the decision-making process. The constant development of new knowledge to support decisions will also help.

Some practitioners may study for additional formal qualifications, such as a management degree. Even though someone has qualified and registered as a health or social care professional and enjoys the rewards of close contact with service users, after some years of practice a position in management or as a team leader may offer the kind of advancement in a career that is desired. The important thing is to take personal control and to think ahead in terms of what opportunities may arise. This will partially be dictated by the context of practice but will also be influenced by personal circumstances and whether, for example, the employee is free to relocate for employment and career development purposes.

Madill and Hollis (2003) attempted to formulate a picture of advanced practice and to define expertise in the context of health care provision. One definition that was offered, for example, proposed that an advanced practitioner was:

> a professional who has taken active steps to broaden and deepen knowledge of the practice arena in which he or she works ... someone who can demonstrate the ability to operate within the current political, economic, sociological and technological context at a high level of practice in one or more domains, such as education, management, research or clinical work (Madill & Hollis, 2003, p. 32).

Characteristics of those capable of advanced practice might also include:

- understanding the reasons behind what is being done in practice;
- refined levels of critical thinking and analytical skills;
- having well-developed problem-solving skills;
- well-developed skills of teamwork and clinical leadership;
- having ability to deal with a complex caseload;
- having a commitment to quality;
- continually adding to personal knowledge;
- having sophisticated learning skills;
- having ability to examine and evaluate personal effectiveness;
- keeping abreast of current developments in the field;
- knowing how to locate and use research to provide best practice;
- possessing advanced qualifications;
- having a commitment to the development of others through leadership, teaching, supervision, mentorship, professional dialogue and debate.

(See also Alsop, 2003)

The above list of talents may serve as a checklist to assess personal qualities in relation to advanced practice. Therefore, the role of advanced practitioner is likely to have requirements that span practice, leadership, research and education. In the United Kingdom, the role of consultant therapist has been created to reflect these advanced skills. The advanced practitioner/consultant therapist role may also be seen as one that offers self-fulfilment and personal satisfaction in the workplace, but investment in CPD has to be made in order to attain the skills to take on such a role.

Career choices

Practitioners often have to consider two parallel worlds when making career decisions: the professional world and the private world. If, for personal or family reasons, a career move to another location is not possible it should not necessarily prevent advancement in a career. A strong identity with selected aspects of practice and willingness to work and progress to expert status in a given field can bring its own rewards. It is always possible to find challenges and so to develop. Updating and continuing to develop professionally in practice prevents stagnation and avoids offering out-of-date practice. Self-monitoring is key. Taking a critical view of one's own performance, knowledge and skills from time to time can highlight areas where improvement and knowledge enhancement is both possible and desirable. If responsibilities in the private world take preference over opportunities in the professional world alternative strategies for personal and professional development can be adopted. It may be the right time to consider taking a further qualification. A Master's degree or professional doctorate can help develop, not just knowledge of practice, but critical skills and research techniques. Developing theory 'helps us recognise what we know and organise what we do. Theory provides the clarity and necessary guidance for solving complex problems in a fast-paced and increasingly complex world' (Mitcham, 2003, p. 67). Alternatively, a degree such as a Master's in Business Administration (MBA) could help develop complementary skills and so help to prepare for a new role when the opportunity arises. There will be times during a career when the private world will not be so dominant allowing career development to take precedence. Newly developed knowledge and skills may help widen the choice of employment opportunity. Even temporary work can help.

Whilst the vast majority of health and social care practitioners may work for a public organisation providing services in health and/or social care, some practitioners may purposely select a career in private practice. Some professionals may offer assessment and treatment services to members of the general public, often seeing them in their own homes; some practitioners may work in partnerships and in clinics again offering private assessment and treatment services to a wider public. Some may specialise in a selected area of practice, for example in paediatrics. Other specialist practitioners may be employed full or part time by private organisations specialising, for example, in medico-legal work. A growing number of skilled professionals are thus opting out of work in public services and choosing to become self-employed, offering private services in specialist areas of practice. These are experts in their field of work. In the

United Kingdom, and in many other countries, they are still required to be registered with the relevant regulatory body responsible for public protection and so must fulfil all the obligations of those registered, such as completing CPD requirements.

Another area of practice that attracts professionals away from public services is work in a variety of voluntary services or social enterprises. This work tends to be less stable, relying often on sometimes quite haphazard funding arrangements. Nevertheless, practitioners who choose this type of work tend to do so because they are committed to the cause. They are often working as single-handed practitioners without any professional support. Therefore, they have to be self-reliant and self-managing as well as experts in their own field of practice. Certainly in the United Kingdom, even if the title of their position does not indicate their profession, if they have taken the job on the basis of their professional expertise, they too must be registered with the HCPC and must comply with CPD requirements. They must find ways of keeping their expertise up to date, ideally through contact with other practising professionals. All single-handed practitioners should make the effort to keep in contact with other members of their own profession and ideally should be members of their professional body. In order to maintain expertise it is critical that isolated practitioners find ways of learning about any new techniques, and the outcomes of relevant research and advances in practice so that they can update their practice and maintain a satisfactory level of expertise.

Professional isolation

Some people enjoy working single-handed and taking the steps, as necessary, to identify support mechanisms that meet their particular needs as and when required. Working with members of other professions in multi- or inter-disciplinary teams places the focus of support on the collegiality of team members. Each member brings both common and unique skills to the team and that blend of skilled resource serves both team and users of the service very well. The team relationships compensate for any isolation that a sole professional may feel. This assumes cooperation rather than conflict. Conflict occurs when individuals or groups work against each other to realise their own goals where these are mutually incompatible (Pollard et al., 2009). Sometimes, experiencing conflict means challenging the status quo in order to bring about harmony that better serves the collective need. Different perspectives aired and shared may encourage knowledge and skills to develop collectively as well-found expertise is needed to support the service being provided. Advanced practice takes account of alternative learning mechanisms and single-handed experience. However, every practitioner still has a responsibility to ensure that professional development occurs that seeks and takes account of research, new ideas and new ways of working. Sometimes the research may be generated by the team. Otherwise, individual team members have a responsibility to link into professional networks that can help them keep up to date.

However, sometimes a 'team' may be hard to identify so that individual professionals perceive themselves to be working in isolation. Single-handed practitioners could be working in rural areas in many parts of the world, possibly where there is significant deprivation and lack of resources. Newton and Fuller (2005) explained some of the challenges that occupational therapists experienced in rural and remote areas. Limited resources, educational opportunities and professional support could be the norm. Similar situations could be experienced by members of other professions. Those working in developing countries could arguably be more deprived than colleagues practising in more developed areas. Professional isolation could result and could even be exacerbated by political tensions. Wherever possible, steps should be taken to maintain contact with professional colleagues such as through the Occupational Therapy International Outreach Network (OTION) project (Newton & Fuller, 2005) to counter professional isolation. The Occupational Therapy International Outreach Network, otherwise known as OTION, is an internet-based network established to support colleagues working in developing countries and other challenging settings. Established in 2001 by volunteers, the network aims to facilitate the exchange of information and learning and also to help overcome professional isolation. Discussion forums help professionals working in different countries to engage in discussion and to assist with inquiries from colleagues. It is hoped to extend the concept to support members of other professions in due course (Newton & Fuller, 2005). Other social networks can provide a similar service helping to minimise the effects of social isolation and maximise opportunities to keep in touch nationally and internationally with those with similar interests.

Mentoring as an aid to career success

Kelly and Marin (1998) have argued that career success and upward mobility can be enhanced by mentorship, whether in a formal or informal capacity. This is particularly so for women, although there is reason to think that men might also benefit. Apart from the more traditional one-to-one relationship, other forms of social contact can also be helpful. Taking advantage of in-house CPD opportunities such as seminars and thus meeting people who might be influential in promoting change could also provide helpful forms of development. It is as important to keep up to date with organisational trends as with practice issues. Competitive advantage is said to stem from awareness of context so that learning can be planned to meet the changing needs of the organisation both technically and managerially.

Mentoring was addressed in some detail in Chapter 3. However, in promoting both career and organisational effectiveness, Hall (2002) offered some insights into different mentoring strategies. He similarly argued that mentoring could take place within different social relationships, for example, in a group of peers. Newcomers, whether new to the organisation or new to a department could help and support each other, including providing emotional support. This may not stretch an employee as much as a more traditional form of mentoring relationship but does offer a collegial form of support that could maximise the efforts of all involved. Hall also promoted another form of mentoring, that of mentors as co-learners. Given the changing nature of organisations, new types of structures that support staff may need to be designed.

Co-learners learn from each other so that support becomes reciprocal in nature. There may no longer be experts in career strategy given that organisational arrangements change frequently and prohibit a longer term view of career development. Co-learning brings two or more minds together, possibly with different expertise, so each becomes a co-inquirer in the search for meaning and career growth in the midst of turbulent times. Another form of professional support includes that of 'critical companion' (Titchen & McGinley, 2004, p. 111), an experienced facilitator who accompanies a practitioner on an experiential learning journey. The companion serves as a resource and facilitator of learning in order to enhance practice. Commonly any form of mentorship is a non-directive relationship with another person that uses dialogue to facilitate problem-solving, challenge assumptions and promote learning.

Practical steps to career planning and development

Firstly, it is important to have a personal vision of a future career that could ultimately offer satisfaction at work. Having a vision at least sets a direction even if unforeseen circumstances make it difficult to attain. There are always choices. Identifying goals that incrementally can help achieve the kind of employment that is desired can provide the impetus to progress and should indicate the direction that should be taken to gain the desired position in employment. Goals may include gaining appropriate experience in a range of work settings or academic qualifications that are prerequisites for some types of employment. It is important to keep a CV up to date and a portfolio of career experiences, reflections, learning outcomes and skills that have been developed for reference when completing an application form or attending an interview. Having a methodical approach to achieving goals and recording important events and achievements indicates progress and commitment to furthering knowledge and experience. Knowing personal strengths and limitations in the process of advancing practice focuses the mind. It is not possible to be good at everything, so limitations can be acknowledged as strengths are highlighted. It is also important to remember that career history and experiences prior to qualification as a health or social care professional can supplement those skills acquired since qualification and in certain circumstances may provide an edge in an application for a post.

Having a vision of a desired career sets a direction but life circumstances and changes in health or social care management strategies can often challenge the route that has been planned. A new direction may have to be set, so learning to be flexible and having the ability to reconceptualise a career is important. A career has to be managed and may go off course from time to time, but changes offer the opportunity to rethink a career. Sometimes it is necessary to take a career break, for childcare, for example. Sometimes a career break may mean leaving the current employment to undertake a secondment, sabbatical or other educational opportunity, research or a job as a volunteer. Keeping in touch with colleagues during the break is important, as is taking steps to manage and complete CPD requirements for ongoing registration with the regulatory body. Nevertheless, all these experiences bring new skills and possibly new career goals. In whatever way a career is advanced, it is crucial that relevant personal and professional development activities are added to the CV and that the CV is kept up to date as part of a portfolio.

Summary

This chapter has further addressed the concept of career and explored ways in which a career may be approached. It is advocated that work-related activities that underpin career development should be recorded as CPD. Ways of advancing in a career and developing expertise in professional practice are considered. The perceived characteristics of an advanced practitioner are highlighted. Other steps for advancing a career, such as undertaking further academic study are also considered. Many health and social care professionals review their position working for a public organisation and decide on other options for employment such as private practice, work in community practices, voluntary services or social enterprises. Ways in which professional isolation can be managed are addressed with special reference to mentorship and the use of social networks. Suggestions for ways of planning and pursuing a career and attaining personal goals are offered.

References

Alsop A (1992) *The organisation, role and behaviour of occupational therapists in a district general hospital.* Submitted MPhil thesis, University of Bath.

Alsop A (2003) The leading edge of competence: developing your potential for advanced practice. In: *Becoming an Advanced Healthcare Practitioner* (eds G Brown, SA Esdaile & SE Ryan), pp. 260–281. Butterworth-Heinemann, Edinburgh.

Arthur MB, Hall DT & Lawrence BS (1989) Generating new directions in career theory: the case for a transdisciplinary approach. In: *Handbook of Career Theory* (eds MB Arthur, DT Hall & BS Lawrence). Cambridge University Press, Cambridge.

Barnett R (1997) *Higher Education: A Critical Business.* Society for Research into Higher Education and Open University Press, Buckingham.

Beeston S & Higgs J (2001) Professional practice: artistry and connoisseurship. In: *Practice Knowledge and Expertise in the Health Professions* (eds J Higgs & A Titchen), pp. 108–117. Butterworth-Heinemann, Oxford.

Fish D (1998) *Appreciating Practice in the Caring Professions: Refocusing Professional Development and Practitioner Research.* Butterworth-Heinemann, Oxford.

Goulet LR & Singh P (2002) Career commitment: a re-examination and an extension. *Journal of Vocational Behaviour,* **61**, 73–91.

Hall DT (2002) *Careers In and Out of Organisations.* Sage Publications, Thousand Oaks, CA.

Herriot P (1992) *The Career Management Challenge.* Sage Publications, London.

Higgs J (2003) Do you reason like a health professional? In: *Becoming an Advanced Healthcare Practitioner* (eds G Brown, SA Esdaile & SE Ryan), pp. 145–160. Butterworth-Heinemann, Edinburgh.

Higgs J, Andresen L & Fish D (2004a) Practice knowledge – its nature, sources and contexts. In: *Developing Practice Knowledge for Health Professionals* (eds J Higgs, B Richardson & MA Dahlgren), pp. 51–69. Butterworth-Heinemann, Oxford.

Higgs J, Fish D & Rothwell R (2004b) Practice knowledge – critical appreciation. In: *Developing Practice Knowledge for Health Professionals* (eds J Higgs, B Richardson & MA Dahlgren), pp. 89–105. Butterworth-Heinemann, Oxford.

Kelly RM & Marin AJD (1998) Position power and women's career advancement. *Women in Management Review*, **13** (2), 53–66.

Madill H & Hollis V (2003) Developing competencies for advanced practice: how do I get there from here? In: *Becoming an Advanced Healthcare Practitioner* (eds G Brown, SA Esdaile & SE Ryan), pp. 30–63. Butterworth-Heinemann, Edinburgh.

Mitcham MD (2003) Integrating theory and practice: using theory creatively to enhance professional practice. In: *Becoming an Advanced Healthcare Practitioner* (eds G Brown, SA Esdaile & SE Ryan), pp. 64–89. Butterworth-Heinemann, Edinburgh.

Newton E & Fuller B (2005) The Occupational Therapy International Outreach Network: supporting occupational therapists working without borders. In: *Occupational Therapy Without Borders: Learning from the Spirit of Survivors* (eds F Kronenberg, S Simó Algado & N Pollard), pp. 361–373. Elsevier Churchill Livingstone, Edinburgh.

Pollard N, Sakellariou D & Kronenberg F (2009) Political competence in occupational therapy. In: *Political Practice of Occupational Therapy* (eds N Pollard, D Sakellariou & F Kronenberg), pp. 21–38. Churchill Livingstone, Edinburgh.

Schein EH (1978) *Career Dynamics: Matching Organisational and Individual Needs*. Addison-Wesley, Reading, MA.

Titchen A & McGinley M (2004) Blending self-knowledge and professional knowledge in person-centred care. In: *Developing Practice Knowledge for Health Professionals* (eds J Higgs, B Rihardson & MA Dahlgren), pp. 107–126. Butterworth-Heinemann, Oxford.

Whymark K & Ellis S (1999) Whose career is it anyway? Options for career management in flatter organisational structures. *Career Development International*, **4** (2), 117–120.

Woodd M (2000) The psychology of career theory – a new perspective?. *Career Development International*, **5** (6), 273–278.

Yarnall J (1998) Career anchors: results of an organisational study in the UK. *Career Development International*, **3** (2), 56–61.

Chapter 11

CPD and career development for academics

This chapter addresses:

1. the common experience of practising professionals who assume a role in academia;
2. ways of developing a career and improving teaching practices in the academic environment;
3. continuing professional development (CPD) opportunities for those working in an academic setting.

Introduction

Those health and social care professionals who work in institutions of higher education are likely to have access to a range of learning opportunities that might be considered as continuing professional development (CPD). One of the key challenges for lecturers who must fulfil the requirements of a regulatory body such as the Health and Care Professions Council (HCPC) is to demonstrate how the CPD activities undertaken might impact positively on service users. Lecturers tend primarily to be associated with students of their profession, although different roles can take them into practice and into contact with service personnel and occasionally with service users. Some lecturers prefer to maintain an active role in practice through part-time work so that their practice informs their academic work and vice versa. This pattern of work can have costs and benefits for the individual and for employers. However, many would argue that the benefits outweigh the disadvantages by continuing to provide opportunities for contact with services. Some health professionals become self-employed and develop independent practice for part of the working week and thus maintain their contact with service users and some control over that aspect of their work. The challenge for all practitioners, whether in practice or in academia, is to find the time to develop and maintain a portfolio, which includes records of all significant learning events that are pertinent to CPD, and that shows links with

Continuing Professional Development in Health and Social Care: Strategies for Lifelong Learning, Second Edition. Auldeen Alsop.
© 2013 John Wiley & Sons, Ltd. Published 2013 by John Wiley & Sons, Ltd.

improving practice. Most events will offer opportunities for learning provided that critical reflection on the event takes place.

The early academic career

Most lecturers in the health and social care professions are recruited from practice. In practice, they tend to be experts in their field of work. Most aspiring lecturers are professionals who have already contributed to student education by supervising, teaching and assessing students in the workplace and perhaps lecturing students in the local university. The education of health and social care students is a joint responsibility between universities and the practice environment and there are several ways in which practitioners can become involved in course delivery as preparation for a teaching post. Being involved with student recruitment, curriculum planning, university committee work and validation (university course approval) events are some of the important activities in which practitioners could also be involved with the university. Some practitioners may become involved in supervising student research projects or in collaborating in university practice research projects themselves. Engaging in these activities may lead some practitioners to consider applying for employment within the institution of higher education as a career move with a view to becoming even more involved in student learning and in their own academic and professional development. Although there are variations across the world, lecturers in higher education would not commonly be appointed without a Master's degree, and in some cases a doctorate. Therefore, anyone looking to move from practice to education would need to take advice on the minimum academic qualification required and make an effort first to achieve the necessary qualification.

Surprising as it may seem, it can take a year or more for practitioners to settle into the academic environment. This may seem a long time in order to socialise into a new work setting, but those who have made the transition from practice to academia tend to agree with this expectation. Everything is new, including the language and the rules and regulations that govern the academic programmes. New lecturers need to see the full pattern of the academic year, become conversant with their responsibilities within the teaching team, engage with the lecturing role that often requires significant preparation time in the early days, and they need to learn to meet assessment and feedback deadlines. Newly appointed lecturers, who come from practice where they are experts in their field, admit that they become novices in the academic world as they take on new roles and responsibilities in the university. This requires a degree of patience as the new lecturer adopts the role of learner in the new setting.

Whatever their role in practice, education or research, it is true to say that all professionals are also learners, regardless of the stage of their career, as they learn from colleagues and students, from networking and from self-reflection. An openness to new learning enables best practice in the work environment and such a disposition fosters learning that can be of benefit to the whole community. The more supportive the work environment, the more the community can cope with the challenges that employment in an institution of higher education can bring. If the community of learning is part of a wider learning organisation it should find workable solutions to challenges faced in the academic environment. Constant change within organisations and concern about value for money, efficiencies and reputation are likely to be talking points that have been experienced in practice, but have to be played out in a different way in education. Lecturers are required to be innovative and put forward schemes for income generation at the same time as maintaining the highest standards of education for students. Supporting a learning organisation can set the challenges in context and help positive solutions to be found. The new learning that goes on during the first year of appointment as a lecturer, and beyond that in academia, is considerable. Reflections on different aspects of the process of accommodation within the academic environment are worthy of inclusion in a CPD portfolio.

Teaching qualification

Even though a Master's degree or doctorate may be the minimum qualification for gaining a lecturing position, once employed within the university the next academic award to be undertaken, certainly in the United Kingdom, would need to be a Post-graduate Certificate in Higher Education (PG Cert HE) as a necessary teaching qualification. Those with aspirations to work in higher education might even consider studying for the PG Cert HE whilst still in practice. This would not only place applicants for lecturing posts at an advantage but would also prepare practitioners for developing creative ways of facilitating student learning in the practice environment. The university would normally make provision for new lecturers without this qualification to undertake the course within the university. The course would normally take 1 year, part time, to complete. Any such academic course that is associated with student education can be listed for CPD purposes if the lecturer is targeted for audit by the regulatory body. There is a clear link between studying for the qualification and enhancing student practice to the benefit of service users. Once acclimatised to the work of the university and having achieved any essential qualifications it should then be possible to consider other personal and professional development opportunities, including research. Those working in higher education must still maintain a portfolio of learning from CPD opportunities.

A continuing career in academia

Ongoing work within a university provides opportunities to innovate and to develop teaching, learning and assessment strategies that maximise student potential and prepare them well for practice. Familiarisation with different roles within the academic team and the wider education system also brings new challenges and learning opportunities. For example, a lecturer may additionally take responsibility for recruiting and selecting students for a course, for supporting students with special needs whilst they are undertaking a course, or for visiting students in practice locations. These all demand the development of specialised knowledge and skills for the role. New academic courses have also to be developed and approved periodically and that entails significant extra work for the team. This process would naturally bring lecturers and practitioners together to explore strengths and limitations of any existing course that is subject to periodic review and to determine areas for development within a new course. Courses leading to the professional qualification in the United Kingdom require approval by the HCPC and relevant professional body as well as the university. Similar requirements exist elsewhere in the world so the demands on an academic team developing a new course for approval are not inconsiderable, and in themselves constitute a learning process.

Other learning opportunities come from taking up roles with other universities. The external examiner system is part of a university's quality assurance mechanism. Lecturers with appropriate qualifications and experience from one or more universities are appointed by the host university to appraise the work of its students who are studying for a qualification similar to that held by the visiting lecturer(s). The objective is to support the host university in maintaining its standards of education through evaluation and feedback on the work that is appraised and the quality of the academic programme as a whole. Similarly, a lecturer from one university may be invited to sit on a validation (course approval) panel of another university to assess, as an objective participant, the strengths and limitations of a proposed new course and determine its fitness for the proposed qualification. Lecturers are thus using their expertise within the environment of another university and yet gaining exposure to alternative ways of presenting course material and using learning, teaching and assessment strategies in course delivery.

UK Professional Standards Framework

The UK Professional Standards Framework (UKPSF) (2011) was developed by the Higher Education Academy (HEA) and is presented as a set of statements that outlines the key characteristics of various teaching roles within higher education (www.heacademy.ac.uk/ukpsf; accessed 25 September 2012). The HEA is an independent organisation in the United Kingdom that supports those working in higher education with the aim of enhancing the quality and impact of learning and teaching. The UKPSF is intended to assist institutions to support the initial and continuing professional development of staff who are engaged in teaching and in supporting and facilitating learning. The framework claims to foster dynamic approaches to teaching and learning through creativity, innovation and continuous development in order to improve the quality of teaching practice. The underpinning expectation is that lecturers will engage in CPD activity that enhances their teaching capability as well as their practice knowledge. Teaching capability includes the design and planning of learning programmes and activities, ways of teaching and supporting learning, assessing and giving feedback and developing effective learning environments and approaches to student guidance and support. It encourages the development of appropriate and effective methods for teaching specific subject material with due respect for a range of professional values that acknowledge the learner, the use of scholarship and the wider context of professional practice.

The framework also helps define the career stages of academic personnel from staff new to teaching to those with more teaching experience and extended roles in higher education or practice settings. From there, the framework addresses the expectations of experienced staff who take on leadership roles and finally the more senior staff with wide-ranging academic and/or strategic roles. For health and social care professionals working in higher education, the framework provides for career development and indicates the expectations of those working at the different career stages. The framework thus provides a reference for professionals as they maintain their CV, their professional portfolio and respond to the HCPC audit.

Keeping in touch with practice

Educators are commonly accused by practitioners of being out of touch with practice as their teaching appears to focus increasingly on theory and its application rather than on the practical aspects of practice. Educators, of course, argue that they have a responsibility to ensure that students meet the standards of education as laid down by the regulatory body, the professional body and the university and these include the application of both theory and practice. Nevertheless, it is a responsibility of educators to make sure they have credibility amongst their peers in practice by undertaking activities and having commitments that bring them into contact with practice. Responsibilities that extend to practice provide opportunities for association with services and so have direct or indirect links with service users. These activities could well be used as evidence of CPD provided that new learning is identified. For example, some of the ways in which it is possible to keep in touch with practice and so maintain and update practice skills are as follows:

- Visiting students in practice situations.
- Attending and contributing to team meetings in a designated service.
- Attending and contributing to joint CPD initiatives between service and academic personnel.
- Undertaking a secondment in practice.
- Having a part-time work commitment in practice.
- Experiencing a job exchange with someone in practice.
- Job-sharing with someone based in practice.
- Undertaking a collaborative research project with a practitioner.
- Supporting/supervising practitioners who are undertaking practice-related research.
- Attending conference sessions that focus on practice.
- Collaborating with practitioners in the preparation of a practice-related article for publication.
- Becoming a member of a Board or Committee of the Professional Body where practice is discussed.

Active engagement with any of these experiences could help maintain practice knowledge and support teaching activity. Directly or indirectly, academic staff must be able to demonstrate that some of their CPD opportunities benefit service users. Creative initiatives that allow contact with practice can help demonstrate that professional updating is occurring that has direct relevance to practice and to service users. Indirectly, research and learning that supports teaching, including reading and critically appraising journal articles, will benefit students and through them should benefit service users. It is up to the academic staff member to keep records of these learning opportunities and to make the connection between the learning and, indirectly, the benefit or potential benefit to service users.

Service learning and community engagement

In many countries, the whole ethos of health and social care is changing. There is a shift of responsibility away from institutional health and social care towards community-based rehabilitation and health promotion initiatives with individuals and communities. These initiatives encourage active participation of individuals and communities as agents of change to promote their own health and well-being. It is not unusual for university staff and students to co-operate with such schemes as a social responsibility. Whilst these offer ad hoc learning opportunities, those initiatives that are designated as 'service learning' initiatives are purposely established as learning environments by the community and university. Service learning has been defined as:

> A strategy through which students engage with a community so they learn and develop together through organised service that meets mutually identified needs. Service learning helps foster civic responsibility through coordinated activity with a higher education institution and a community. It is an integral part of the academic curriculum (which may be credit-bearing) and includes structured time for role players ... to reflect on the service experience and modify actions if indicated (Lorenzo et al., 2006, p. 276).

Service learning initiatives are known to operate in the United States and South Africa with students of many disciplines involved, and not just those from health and social care. Other schemes may be in their infancy. Pritchard (2001) distinguished between community service and service learning by suggesting that service learning:

- has clearly defined objectives;
- expects student involvement in selecting or designing the service activity;
- has a theoretical base;
- integrates the service experience with the academic curriculum;
- offers opportunity for student reflection.

Compared with practice learning, service-learning initiatives offer a learning context for all parties, and not just students. University staff are normally instrumental in locating relevant service learning sites and establishing the working arrangements between the site and the university. Ultimately, students may be responsible for negotiating entry to the site, engaging with community members to agree and undertake a project or scheme of work and for the planned withdrawal from the experience under the terms of the scheme. Academic staff support the learning by ensuring that objectives are met, students have the opportunity for reflection and that work is set in a theoretical context, as relevant to the curriculum. These initiatives extend the university into the community and offer opportunities for academic staff to have direct contact with service users. These initiatives are collaborative learning schemes that serve the needs of all participants in different ways. As far as lecturers are concerned, schemes such as service learning and other community projects enable them to take their expertise to service users and then show how their efforts could be of benefit. Reflections on such initiatives can be recorded as CPD.

Other CPD opportunities

Academic staff tend to have many opportunities to develop their knowledge, skills and practices provided that they can justify taking advantage of those opportunities as part of their academic role. This also means ensuring that students are not disadvantaged by the time taken to undertake the CPD initiative and that in fact students may well benefit directly or indirectly from it. Apart from the initiatives listed above, other opportunities may present themselves. The most obvious is attendance at relevant conferences, although financial support for this normally depends on the academic having prepared a poster or verbal presentation for the conference or on being an invited speaker. These preparations are equally important for CPD as they require research and critical decisions about their presentation and application. The number of conference opportunities, both nationally and internationally, is many and varied, so it is often necessary to be selective. There are also likely to be financial limitations making selectivity essential. Conferences provide opportunities for both formal and informal discussions with colleagues that often lead to collaborations on other projects and the potential for exchange visits. Learning about research that is being undertaken and new practices that are being evaluated can be of enormous benefit. Making comparisons between practices in different services and different countries can open eyes to new ways of working. The 'twinning' of universities in different countries that offer similar professional qualification programmes could bring opportunities for academic development through exchange lecturing programmes or collaboration or dissemination of research. Again, these events can be documented as CPD that indicates learning.

Some universities offer schemes to staff that allow sabbaticals after a specified period of employment. Sabbaticals must normally have a clear professional development plan with approved outcomes to be achieved in an agreed length of time. Although there may be some financial implications for the academic's salary, the gains to be achieved through the development opportunity can outweigh the financial drawback. Some people take a sabbatical to finalise a PhD thesis. Others might look to explore research opportunities at home or abroad. The freedom that a sabbatical allows presents the opportunity to travel and expand horizons, possibly by exploring or contributing to practice in other countries. From time to time, sponsorships or grants may be offered for research or other activities associated with specific projects. These are normally obtained through competitive application and have expectations that must be met within a given timeframe. The sponsorship, if won, will cover travel, accommodation and/or activities as specified by the sponsor, up to a defined maximum amount. Often academic departments are circulated with information about relevant sponsorships, although individuals may also seek them out privately.

There are also scholarships to be won. For example, there are Commonwealth scholarships and academic and professional fellowship schemes that support career development opportunities for professionals (see, e.g., www.britishcouncil.org; www.csfp-online.org) The CPD opportunity can come as much from hosting an extended visit from a professional from a developing or other country within the Commonwealth as from applying to undertake the scholarship personally. Websites in the Commonwealth countries will provide relevant information about the application process and expectations. The host organisation normally has to make the application to participate in the scheme, and receive and make necessary provision for the development of the visiting professional, according to his or her interests and the potential benefits to the participant's country of origin. The scheme can be mutually advantageous, with learning occurring on both sides.

European schemes also exist to support the professional development of academics. For example, the Grundtvig scheme designed to promote innovation and creativity in adult education through enhanced trans-national cooperation offers opportunities for academics to apply for grants from the European Commission to attend work-related training courses to improve knowledge and skills. The focus is on promoting staff mobility across Europe and supporting learning partnerships between institutions in European countries (www.ec.europa.eu/education/lifelong-learning-programme/grundtvig_en.htm; accessed 26 September 2012).

Professional bodies may also have links with World Federations or European schemes that promote engagement with initiatives for the advancement of knowledge and practice. For example, the European Network of Occupational Therapy in Higher Education (ENOTHE; www.enothe.eu) is a thematic network that has financial support from the ERASMUS scheme of the European Commission. The aim is to enhance quality in education and to define a European dimension within an academic discipline. A similar initiative exists for social workers – the European Platform for Worldwide Social Work (EUSW). Both ENOTHE and EUSW are part of the Archipelago of the Humanistic Thematic Networks that address aspects of the Humanistic Arts and Sciences (see http://www.archhumannets.net). These schemes offer professionals opportunities to contribute to initiatives that advance practice and participate in wider European development opportunities that promote collaboration and learning.

Research

Ronald Barnett (1997, 2000, 2003) has long questioned the purpose of the university in modern society and the role of academics within them. In earlier work, Barnett

(1994) stressed the importance of professional legitimacy and advocated that one responsibility of professionals was to shape change and thus remain competent in an ever-changing world. New knowledge and practices had to replace old ones but in advancing this notion professionals had to become knowledge creators. In the light of this, Barnett (1997, p. 140) saw professionals as *practising epistemologists*, 'able to interpret the world through cognitive frameworks and be adept at handling those frameworks in action'. This required professionals to become proficient at critical thinking and not just at problem-solving in professional situations. Undertaking research, or at least engaging seriously with evidence that is pertinent to practice, must therefore be high on a professional's agenda. However, Cusick (2001) acknowledged the challenges that practitioners experience in trying to carry out research in practice. However, she also maintained that there were possibilities for collaboration suggesting that academic researchers became the partners of practitioners for the purpose of research. These sorts of collaborations should enable both practitioners and academics to engage in purposeful research not only as a CPD activity but also for enabling the professions to add to their body of practice knowledge.

Given that most academics emerge from having worked in practice situations, it could be suggested that at least some newly appointed university lecturers aspire to be knowledge creators interested in developing their capacity for research. Some may see the university as an institution that would support PhD studies (or even post-doctoral research) in order to boost both the university's research profile and the qualifications and CVs of the staff. However, the reality of work pressures in a university has to be discovered before research interests can be realised unless, of course, the university appointment specifies research expectations. Barnett (2005) commented on the many and varied expectations of teaching staff over and above their teaching commitments as 'suffocating' in the new era of income-focused universities. There was a clear need to sort out the relationships between teaching and research and thus the responsibilities of staff where there was an expectation of best practice in both domains.

Maggie Savin-Baden (2008) acknowledged from her own academic experience that it was difficult to find what she termed 'spaces' for her own professional development in the academic environment. She captured the essence of what many academics feel to be the challenges in academia. She suggested that lecturers are now overwhelmed by mundane administrative duties and thus denied the time and space to engage in the more creative, academic activities of thinking, reflecting, reading, writing and engaging in research. She intimated that finding and using space for knowledge creation was little valued by universities and that this had to change if universities were to reposition themselves in the world of intellectual thought. It was thus important to find ways of protecting personal 'spaces' that could be used more productively for developing ideas and transforming them into meaningful academic outcomes for the benefit of society that included the academic and practice world. Of course, other collaborators in research could involve service users and groups of people in the community that represent service users and promote their needs and expectations. Joint research between community support groups or community action groups and academics in the health and social care professions can really make a difference in practice.

There is no doubt that there needs to be more clarity about the expectations of lecturers and their managers with regard to research. Yet we have to assume, based on the history of universities, that research endeavour is both expected and welcomed within the academic setting. Time for different aspects of work in academia may need to be negotiated but if professionals in health and social care are to ensure that their practice is up to date and forging forward with validated new ways of working then engagement with formal research is a necessity and not an option. Fulfilling the CPD requirements becomes a planned benefit of the research activity.

Summary

This chapter has considered the role of professionals who are appointed as lecturers in an institution of higher education and ways in which they can undertake continuing professional development (CPD). Additional academic qualifications such as a Master's degree and teaching qualification may initially be required for the position. The newly appointed academic often finds it challenging to adjust to the roles, responsibilities and work environment of a university lecturer. However, many different CPD opportunities may present themselves, so allowing lecturers to enhance their teaching skills as well as their professional expertise and research skills, and thus the quality of students' learning. Lecturers in the health and social care professions should also endeavour to maintain some contact with service provision. Therefore, various ways of engaging with service users are explored. Opportunities for participating in international development programmes are noted. The responsibilities of academics with regard to engaging in research and in promoting the development of their profession are highlighted, as are the challenges that are sometimes faced by those who aspire to undertaking research.

References

Barnett R (1994) *The Limits of Competence: Knowledge, Higher Education and Society*. The Society for Research into Higher Education and Open University Press, Buckingham.

Barnett R (1997) *Higher Education: A Critical Business*. The Society for Research into Higher Education and Open University Press, Buckingham.

Barnett R (2000) *Realizing the University in an Age of Supercomplexity*. The Society for Research into Higher Education and Open University Press, Buckingham.

Barnett R (2003) *Beyond All Reason: Living with Ideology in the University*. The Society for Research into Higher Education and Open University Press, Buckingham.

Barnett R (ed.) (2005) *Reshaping the University: New Relationships Between Research, Scholarship and Teaching*. The Society for Research into Higher Education and Open University Press, Buckingham.

Cusick A (2001) The research sensitive practitioner. In: *Professional Practice in Health, Education and the Creative Arts* (eds J Higgs & A Titchen), pp. 125–135. Blackwell Science, Oxford.

Lorenzo T, Duncan M, Buchanan H & Alsop A (eds) (2006) *Practice and Service Learning in Occupational Therapy: Enhancing Potential in Context*. John Wiley & Sons, Chichester.

Pritchard IA (2001) Community service and service-learning in America: the state of the art. In: *Service-Learning the Essence of the Pedagogy* (eds A Furco & SH Billig), pp. 3–21. Information Age Publishing, Greenwich, CT.

Savin-Baden M (2008) *Learning Spaces: Creating Opportunities for Knowledge Creation in Academic Life*. The Society for Research into Higher Education and Open University Press, Buckingham.

Chapter 12

Leadership and professional development

This chapter addresses:

1. some perceived differences between leaders and managers;
2. common attributes of a leader;
3. management development and leadership development programmes, mechanisms of support, innovation through leadership and the development of expert practice.

Introduction

The need to take personal responsibility for continuing professional development (CPD) applies to all health and social care practitioners registered with a regulatory body irrespective of position held within the employing organisation or as a private practitioner. So far, chapters in this book have addressed CPD from the perspectives of health and social care professionals with different roles, including those working in academia. This chapter explores the development needs of those holding management or leadership positions within an organisation or those aspiring to become leaders in their profession. Most professionals qualified to work in health or social care will consider their current employment as a stage in their career. Some may be content to work at practitioner level indefinitely, whilst others may aspire to developing their career to take on responsibility for leading teams or managing services. Some practitioners will be identified by their peers or by their managers as having leadership potential. Using such mechanisms as performance review, these practitioners can be incrementally guided towards assuming responsibilities within the service that allow them to develop as leaders.

No matter how many texts are consulted, there appears to be no common definition of leadership, as Yukl (1998) concluded:

> Leadership has been defined in different ways, but most definitions share the assumption that it involves a social influence process whereby intentional influence is exerted by

Continuing Professional Development in Health and Social Care: Strategies for Lifelong Learning, Second Edition. Auldeen Alsop.

one person over other people in an attempt to structure the activities and relationships in a group or organisation (Yukl, 1998, p. 14).

Yukl's observation perceives leadership as a process and this perception appears to be shared by Northouse (2001) who proposed a simplified definition:

Leadership is a process whereby an individual influences a group of individuals to achieve a common goal (Northouse, 2001, p. 2).

Leaders, it seems, make a difference by achieving outcomes that, but for their intervention, would not otherwise have occurred. Put simply, leaders add value to organisational performance (Gronn, 1999) and are thus necessary within organisational structures.

Yukl (1998) also considered the perceived differences between managers and leaders and again there seemed to be differences of opinion. He summed up some of the arguments by suggesting that managers are likely to be oriented towards stability whereas leaders would be oriented towards innovation. He followed that observation with a proposal that managers seek efficiency whereas leaders seek agreement about what needs to be done. Nanus and Dobbs (1999) viewed leaders as those who are concerned with building a future for the organisation where more divergent thinking is required to seek new directions and shape the organisation for the longer term. Although health and social care organisations have a managerial structure, there appears to be an expectation that leadership skills should be developed at all levels of the organisation. However, as is noted below, different ways of thinking and working may be required of the two roles.

Management development

Given the more typical hierarchical structure of health and social care organisations, those who head up teams or services are likely to be designated as managers. It could be argued that the term manager is usually associated with the management of various resources such as human, financial or other physical resources. These resources must be deployed efficiently and effectively in order to meet the goals of the organisation. The responsibility and accountability for completing delegated tasks to a satisfactory standard within available resources normally rests with managers. Some practitioners who seek management positions may elect to complete an academic award such as a Master's in Business Administration (MBA) to assist them with understanding the nature of activities that they may be asked to perform. Those who are appointed as managers may otherwise be offered in-service training and/or mentorship and will otherwise be supervised by their line manager as they develop their skills in the art of management. It is commonly believed these days that health and social care professionals should have education and training in management techniques as increasingly health and social care provision is seen as a business requiring the use of business 'thinking' and business skills. The better the understanding of the business, the more focused will managers be on the goals that have to be achieved.

Those allied health professionals who have independent businesses or practices will have a management role, although their title might be Director or Consultant. They may have leadership qualities but their activities are business oriented. However, it is equally essential for them to maintain and develop their practice skills and expertise with relevant CPD activity as they, too, will be subject to audit by the regulatory body. CPD may emerge from undertaking research, formal qualifications, from designated in-service training, from case studies or from project work associated with the role of practitioner, manager or leader.

Leadership

For the most part, leadership is not thought of as the same as management, although good leadership skills may be considered an asset for those in management positions. Nanus and Dobbs (1999) viewed managing and leading as quite different functions requiring separate mindsets and different skills. Managers, they claimed, must focus on what needs to be done and how it can be accomplished within a budget whereas leaders are more concerned with strategy and direction, particularly for the longer term, and in securing the growth of the organisation. If leadership is about setting a direction for others to follow and influencing the way in which a common and future goal is achieved then those who are considered to be leaders must possess attributes that facilitate this process.

Attributes of a leader

In general, leaders have been described as possessing some or all of the following qualities:

- Clear vision and strategy.
- The ability to listen and communicate the vision to others.
- Ability to take responsibility, take decisions and take and manage risk.
- Self-confidence, knowledge of own strengths and limitations.
- Clear values.
- Positive regard for self and others.
- The ability to motivate people and encourage individual contribution.
- The courage to challenge the status quo and the skills and confidence to offer viable alternatives.
- The ability to deal with uncertainty.
- Team-building skills and an ability to maintain cohesiveness.
- Entrepreneurial skills and the ability to innovate.
- Facilitation skills.
- Skills that promote problem-solving.
- The ability to make effective judgements.
- Skills to manage and resolve conflict and deal with crises.
- Skills of change management.
- Enjoyment of lifelong learning.

The art of leading sometimes includes knowing when to lead and when to hold back and allow others to take control. Delegating and being supportive of others in their ideas and actions is similarly a part of the leadership role. Some theorists consider leadership skills and abilities to be innate others believe they can be developed. It is possible to self-assess and determine personal strengths and limitations using this list as a guide. However, more often than not, colleagues know intuitively when they have a leader in their midst. They make their own judgement about a person's leadership potential. Those leaders who seem to have a natural tendency towards leading and innovating are often perceived by their peers to be inspirational leaders. They have a knack of seeing where change could be beneficial and have the skills and personality to encourage others to bring about that change. Leadership development programmes are available to support other aspiring leaders. Testing out the skills in practice, that is, by experiential learning and reflection on personal performance in a leadership capacity, can equally (if not better) assist in developing knowledge of personal strengths and limitations as a leader.

Leadership development

In the recent past, in the United Kingdom, there has been significant emphasis on the development of leadership skills for all those working in health or social care settings, irrespective of their position within the organisation. As opposed to management development, the focus on leadership development was thought to bring a sense of purpose to the work and enable individuals both to act confidently in their own role and to contribute effectively to teamwork and thus bring a sense of ownership to the tasks in which they engage. In the NHS, leadership development has evolved over time from development courses requiring face-to-face contact to e-learning programmes that individuals can work through at their own pace, such as the Leadership Development Module set within the Leadership Framework that can be accessed at any time (http://nhsleadershipframework.rightmanagement.co.uk; accessed 29 April 2012). The framework advocates the 5E approach to development:

Examine – what you want to develop
Experience – relevant activities on the job to promote learning
Exposure – to other ways of acting and learning from others
Education – through training, reading, attending lectures to supplement experience
Evaluate the effectiveness of what you have done.

The Leadership Development Module comprises a number of sub-units that guide learning. These are labelled as following:

- Demonstrating personal qualities
- Working with others
- Managing services
- Improving services
- Setting direction

- Creating the vision
- Delivering the strategy

These sub-units reflect the tasks of a leader as viewed in the United Kingdom by the NHS and are aimed at those working in health and care services irrespective of their discipline or role in the organisation. Each of the sub-units is divided into a number of stages and requires the active participation of the learner. The tasks are practical and the expectation is that tasks will be followed up with reflection on what has transpired.

Organisations have the responsibility to identify and develop potential leaders through a range of creative mechanisms, providing support for those in leadership positions and enabling leadership skills of individuals to be harnessed within the organisation. Good leadership development encourages:

- experimentation;
- reflection;
- critical evaluation;
- knowledge importation;
- information sharing;
- diffusion of knowledge;
- systems thinking.

Evidence of developing and using these skills in practice should be recorded in a journal or portfolio, together with reflections on their actual, or potential, impact on practice.

It could thus be argued that those who support leadership development expect to see a raised level of confidence in all the team members and in the team's ability to collaborate and generate innovative ideas, achieve goals and determine new ways forward. The effective leader would have a clear vision of what needed to be achieved by the team and would be able to convey that to colleagues. Team members would each know their strengths and limitations and contribute to achieving the desired outcome by 'leading' on some part of the initiative and being content 'to follow' on others, according to their skills. Team commitment, good judgement and a common drive to see a project through satisfactorily would demonstrate leadership skills in use. Reflecting on processes and outcomes with a mentor may help capture the learning that has taken place and any further development needs.

Transition to leader

The transition from team member to team leader may be exciting but can also be challenging. The change may only be temporary if taking responsibility for a project with a defined lifespan, but this short-term experience can offer the chance to test personal aptitude for this type of role. It can involve a subtle change in relationships with colleagues, whether it be a temporary measure or a more permanent arrangement as a result of a promotion. The move to a leadership role can also offer the opportunity to demonstrate personal strengths and discover any limitations that might be worth addressing for the future. Taking a leadership role can also be a stressful activity, so mentorship can help explore dynamics and challenges. Keeping a journal of the experience and noting reflections on the ups and downs of project leadership could offer insights into the dynamics of relationships and the relative success of the various aspects of the project. Any personal or professional development needs will be revealed but successes should also be recorded.

Leadership may be thought of as the process wherein an individual influences:

- the interpretation of events;
- the choice of strategies;
- the organisation of work activities;
- the motivation of people to achieve the goals;
- the maintenance of cooperative relationships;
- the development of skills and confidence of members;
- the progression of projects to completion;
- the overall development of professional or inter-professional teams and services.

Conversations with a mentor on some of the more challenging processes may help clarify the extent to which the leadership role has been effective. Recording examples in a journal or portfolio of how the process has been used, referring to the bullet points above as a guide, would provide evidence of professional developmental activity. Reflections on the activity may illustrate new learning and future development needs.

Supporting aspiring leaders

There is a responsibility to develop the skills of those who aspire to become leaders or who show leadership potential even though they may not yet believe for themselves that they have the ability. Providing mentorship is one of the key ways of offering support to aspiring leaders. A mentor can help highlight strengths and limitations that may not immediately be recognised by the mentee. For example, learning to delegate to team members is a crucial aspect of leadership. The leader cannot undertake all tasks bound up with a project so must appreciate how to make the most of the skills that other team members offer. It requires confidence to 'let go' of actions and to have trust in others that they will complete the task. A clear time frame has to be given along with any guidance and support that appears relevant. A mentor can enable a mentee to see ways of problem-solving as well as prompt the mentee to reflect on the relative success of decisions ultimately made. Mentors can help leaders to flourish but it also has to be noted that those who help develop leaders, such as mentors, are also learning through taking on such a role. Mentorship becomes a CPD activity.

Leadership development and action learning

Leadership courses can help aspiring leaders to learn about some of the scenarios that leaders face. Case studies introduced into the training can illustrate common leadership challenges and encourage debate on ways of addressing the issues. Experiential learning is really the only way of gaining a true insight into the role, including dealing with some of the emotional challenges and difficult decisions that present themselves. Yukl (1998) suggested that it was essential for those in leadership development to experience success in handling difficult challenges as it helped them to develop new skills and self-confidence. Also, the experience of tackling a variety of assignments helps build skills. Secondments, rotating responsibilities between potential leaders and delegating specific assignments can offer opportunities for the novice leader, supported wherever possible with mentorship. Providing feedback on all activities and decisions is important.

One way commonly used to help develop leaders in their role is action learning, a technique developed by Revens (1982). Action learning has been deemed a process of inquiry particularly suited to mature individuals who are willing to deal openly with conflict and challenge in a group where diverse and disparate perspectives may be openly discussed (Herasymowych & Senko, 2000). The group comprises 6–8 members who agree to meet regularly over a period of several months and who are prepared to explore complex organisational problems. Sometimes a skilled facilitator is appointed to work with the group (Yukl, 1998), although some groups may be self-supporting and operate without a facilitator.

At the first meeting, ground rules are set so that the group can function effectively. These include agreeing ethical principles such as maintaining confidentiality and not relaying group discussions outside of the group. There may also be rules that determine how contributions to discussions are made and respect for the views of others. The group then decides on the problem to be discussed. Real-life problems are brought to the group by its members and the group decides on the specific problem to be addressed. The 'problem owner' then tells the group about the issue in more depth. Other members of the group then ask questions but avoid offering advice or solutions at this stage. The problem owner then restates the issue after which possible solutions are generated by the group. The problem owner can decide on which of the alternatives might be pursued (Herasymowych & Senko, 2000). This briefly describes the process. Yukl (1998) observed that unless the project involves considerable challenge it is unlikely to lead to much learning. Additionally, the skills that are developed are more likely to be cognitive and interpersonal skills. However, anecdotally, individuals who have experienced the group process claim that the support of the group is particularly helpful. They often discover that similar problems have been experienced by others who are then able to suggest reasonable strategies for addressing the issue.

Organisational change through leadership

> Leadership . . . is one of the most important elements in achieving change in an organi-
> sation. Leadership sets the vision, direction and tone of the organisation as a whole and
> thus influences the nature and levels of energy, life and commitment in the workforce.
> The focus of any leader should be on the growth and development of the staff so that

they can constantly 'learn to learn', create, innovate and take risks to improve their areas of practice and fulfil the commitment of clinical governance (Chin, 2003, p. 264).

Chin (2003) continued by suggesting that facilitative leadership is based on an ethical commitment to the growth and development of everyone in the organisation.

Innovation

One widely held view is that leaders are often entrepreneurs and innovators. Entrepreneurs tend to be good at weighing up risks and taking projects forward (often successfully) despite any identified risks or challenges. Not everyone is inclined towards high risk, although the ability to manage some element of risk is a necessary function of a leader. Having the capacity to be innovative is another matter. Leaders often emerge because they have a vision of how tasks can be done differently and the ability to inspire others to help create the change. Innovators are creative. They have ideas and actively seek information to support them and use the information wisely to put ideas into action (Rogers, 2003).

Innovators are people who can cope with relatively high levels of uncertainty, are prepared to take risks and have the capacity to bring new ideas into practice. An innovation, according to Rogers (2003), has particular characteristics in that it would normally have a particular advantage over the present situation and be consistent with the values and needs of those for whom it is intended. The degree of complexity, the ability to test out the innovation and the degree to which results are visible to others will often determine how readily an idea might be taken up. Although not everyone will perceive themselves as innovative, Petty (1997) argued that everyone has the ability to be creative, suggesting that in some way or another individuals show their creative side every day. 'Whenever a problem is solved or a difficulty overcome, whenever something new is made or something old adapted, creativity has been at work' (Petty, 1997, p. 13). However, Petty does suggest that some people are creative intuitively whilst others may have to develop the skills.

Creative people know how to generate ideas, choose the right ones and put the ideas into operation. Leaders may be creative or may recognise and support the creativity of other team members. Leaders can still be innovative in that they see how creative ideas generated by others can be used innovatively in the problem-solving process. Some ideas may be tried and fail, but new knowledge often emerges from failure. Contemporary professional practice takes place in a context of uncertainty so the need for creativity is not only there but is also essential in order to find effective solutions and optimise change (Titchen & Higgs, 2001). For the most part, change will lead to success; however, not all innovations will be successful. Even if changes do not work out, significant learning will have taken place. The important thing is to capture the process and outcome as a record in a journal, possibly as a case study. The record is important as it highlights a change that has been tried and tested with the intention of improving a service in one way or another. Any lessons learned from failure are thus equally important and just as relevant for CPD purposes.

Expert practitioners

Many health and social care practitioners are experts in their field having developed business skills, mastery in their professional practice and sufficient self-confidence to consider offering expert practice privately outside of the more regulated health and social care system. Lifelong learning has still to be a feature of their role as a leader and consultant in their field (Roberts, 2003) as a way of improving their effectiveness, whether working single-handedly or as a partner or an employee in a business or social enterprise. Most private practitioners might seek to attain at least a Master's degree in a relevant field to show evidence of their expertise and to be able to advertise this to potential customers. Those who head up private practices also have a responsibility to facilitate the development of their team of workers in order to ensure that they remain at the leading edge of competence. Those who advise in legal cases need to keep up to date with the law as well as their practice expertise. Undertaking research is another relevant form of CPD, although this may have financial implications for those reliant on a salary from their own business.

Some expert practitioners may look to extend the scope of their practice by becoming expert in techniques that complement their own practice so as to widen their repertoire of skills and to be able to offer selected clients a more comprehensive service. However, as Roberts (2003) points out, extended scope of practice often means extending one's own practice by developing new areas of skill and expertise normally associated with another profession. Some regulatory bodies have considered the potential of noting areas of extended practice against a practitioner's name on the appropriate Register. However, despite investigations into the implications of this practice, most regulatory bodies have to date resisted the proposal. The scope of practice of a profession remains that which is covered by the approved academic qualifying curriculum of the named profession. The UK Health and Care Professions Council does not prohibit professionals from developing their scope of practice into new areas. However, professionals who do extend the scope of their practice must demonstrate that they have the necessary skills, knowledge and experience to be able to practise lawfully, safely and effectively in the new area of practice and do not pose any danger to themselves or the public. CPD activity must support practice in the new area. In April 2012, the HCPC announced that it would annotate its Register to show where a registrant from the professions of physiotherapy, chiropody/podiatry or radiography had completed an HCPC approved programme in supplementary prescribing (HPC, 2012). Other regulatory bodies internationally may follow in due course and record selected additional qualifications of members that extend their practice, thus providing relevant information about expertise to the general public.

Summary

This chapter has explored perceived differences between leadership and management and highlighted innovation as a particular strength of leaders. Common characteristics of leaders have been indicated. Consideration has been given to the nature of professional development available to managers and leaders, stressing the responsibility of the organisation for providing both development opportunities and support for those aspiring to management and leadership positions. Particular reference has been made to the challenges faced by those placed temporarily in leadership positions. Action learning, as a particularly useful support mechanism for leaders, has been explained. Some practitioners with management or leadership qualities may choose to create private practices and so extend the scope of their work beyond employment within an organisation. The ongoing need for continuing professional development (CPD) has been indicated.

References

Chin H (2003) Achieving change. In: *Clinical Governance and Best Value* (eds S Pickering & J Thompson), pp. 247–274. Churchill Livingstone, Edinburgh.

Gronn P (1999) *The Making of Educational Leaders*. Cassell, London.

Herasymowych M & Senko H (2000) *Solving Real Problems in Real Time: Action Learning Fieldbook*. MHA Institute Inc Publication, Calgary.

HPC (2012) Independent prescribing for physiotherapists and chiropodists/podiatrists. *HPC*, Issue 40, 5. http://www.hpc-uk.org/assets/documents/10003A1AHPCInFocus-Issue40.pdf (accessed 27 September 2012).

Nanus B & Dobbs SM (1999) *Leaders Who Make a Difference*. Jossey-Bass, San Francisco, CA.

Northouse PG (2001) *Leadership Theory and Practice*, 2nd edn. Sage Publications, Thousand Oaks, CA.

Petty R (1997) *How to be Better at Creativity*. The Industrial Society, London.

Revens RW (1982) *The Origins and Growth of Action Learning*. Chatwell-Bratt, Hunt.

Roberts GR (2003) Consultancy and advanced teaming: promoting practice beyond the healthcare environment. In: *Becoming an Advanced Healthcare Practitioner* (eds G Brown, SA Esdaile & SE Ryan), pp. 282–299. Butterworth-Heinemann, Oxford.

Rogers EM (2003) *Diffusion of Innovations*, 5th edn. Free Press, New York.

Titchen A & Higgs J (2001) Towards professional artistry and creativity in practice. In: *Professional Practice in Health, Education and the Creative Arts* (eds J Higgs & A Titchen), pp. 273–290. Blackwell Science, Oxford.

Yukl G (1998) *Leadership in Organisations*, 4th edn. Prentice Hall, Upper Saddle River, NJ.

Chapter 13

Learning strategies and CPD for support workers

This chapter addresses:

1. the rationale for support workers to engage in continuing professional development (CPD);
2. ways of progressing to meet personal development aspirations;
3. factors to be considered if seeking a university place to gain a professional qualification.

Introduction

The need for regulation of support workers, rehabilitation workers and assistants working with regulated health and social care professionals appears still to be a matter of debate. The generic term of support worker will be used for expedience here, although it is recognised that many different job titles might fall into this category. One of the reasons given for not regulating support workers is the degree of risk that their work entails. Support workers tend to be supervised in their role by qualified professionals and therefore the potential for harm to clients is perceived as smaller than that calculated for professionally qualified staff. Nevertheless, support workers are generally expected to abide by ethical principles in the same way as qualified professionals working in health and social care. Some support workers may also be members of a professional organisation and as such are expected to respect the relevant code of ethics and professional conduct associated with that profession. This is currently the position in the United Kingdom. Whilst support workers are not subject to regulation and thus have no mandatory continuing professional development (CPD) requirement, it is erroneous to think that CPD is unnecessary or unhelpful. However, there are places in the world where support workers are regulated or 'certified'. In South Africa, for example, some support workers have always been regulated in the same way as qualified professionals. In countries such as the United States, there are designated examination boards to enable assistant practitioners to gain appropriate

Continuing Professional Development in Health and Social Care: Strategies for Lifelong Learning,
Second Edition. Auldeen Alsop.
© 2013 John Wiley & Sons, Ltd. Published 2013 by John Wiley & Sons, Ltd.

certification and so be recognised by the licensing authorities of the various American states. Ongoing CPD is required to maintain these credentials.

Support workers come from many different backgrounds and have various reasons for seeking this kind of work. Some may see the work as satisfying in its own right without any wish for career progression. Some support workers may already have qualifications such as a degree, for example in psychology or another science, and view support work as a means of using the knowledge gained through that qualification in a constructive way. In contrast, some may be working in such a role to try out the work, to assess their personal suitability for this type of work and to ascertain for themselves, whether to apply for a university place to study for a professional qualification. Regardless of the rationale for undertaking support work there is still a responsibility to pursue some form of development activity in order to maintain skills and use them effectively with clients and in support of professionally qualified colleagues. Support workers must also be responsible for keeping abreast of relevant changes in the nature of health and social care that apply to them and of new approaches to care management to which they contribute. So having established that undertaking CPD is in the best interests of support workers, how should this apply?

Personal expectations and aspirations

Support work in health and social care offers rewarding employment for many people. Whilst one of the primary reasons for CPD is to keep up to date with necessary skills and techniques for health and social care provision, it is not unreasonable to consider personal expectations and aspirations for self-fulfilment and for career development. The employing authority has a responsibility to ensure that individuals undertake mandatory training in those aspects of the work where health and safety is an issue, in order to maintain skills and where new techniques are being introduced. Support workers should keep a record of these training events in a CPD portfolio. Additionally, some employers offer schemes of education to encourage the advancement of support staff in the workplace. National Vocational Qualifications (NVQs) represent one such scheme in the United Kingdom where individuals can follow a relevant educational programme in the workplace for advancement and attainment of a nationally recognised qualification. Each NVQ requires the work of the support worker to be assessed by an authorised assessor to demonstrate that he or she has attained the required competence to fulfil the NVQ requirements. Other countries may have similar schemes, including the US certification scheme as previously mentioned.

More personalised development schemes can be put in place not only for those content in the role they play in service provision but also for those with aspirations to undertake professional education leading to a qualification in one of the health or social care professions. A programme of CPD can be determined through performance review mechanisms and by setting agreed objectives with the line manager. The specific skill areas to be enhanced can be noted and possible ways of developing the skills may be planned. It might also be possible, for example, to arrange for time to be spent with members of other professions or in other departments within or external to the employing organisation to broaden perspectives on health and social care. Inevitably these opportunities will only be offered if the workplace can cope with the absence of the staff member. However, if there is a set of objectives devised that will help the employing department as well as support the advancement of the individual, both interests may well be served. Many types of CPD may be agreed within the parameters of performance review:

- Working alongside professional colleagues in order to develop more advanced skills in a particular area of work.
- Coordination of project work on behalf of the department.
- Time out to read up on health conditions, or scientific or therapeutic techniques.
- Time to participate in in-service study days, workshops or conferences as a representative of the service.
- Time to undertake an Access Course to secure qualifications for entry to higher education.

There are many forms of CPD activity that are relevant to support workers and that can make a significant contribution to service provision as well as enhance the skills of the individual. Personal expectations must also play a part in determining the range and extent of activities that are appropriate for CPD. Specialisation in particular forms of work on behalf of the service can be rewarding. Aspirations to undertake further education to gain a higher academic award or a professional qualification will also guide CPD choices. Engaging with students in the health and social care professions and contributing to their learning whilst in practice can offer insights into the way in which they address their given responsibilities. Those support workers who show interest and potential for advancement will normally be encouraged and sometimes supported to undertake a range of activities that will contribute to the achievement of longer term goals. Performance reviews or appraisals normally provide the opportunity to discuss these aspirations but there is no reason why expectations should not be discussed with the line manager between these reviews, especially if educational opportunities are currently being offered. Clarity can then be gained about what CPD activity the service might support and which activities might have to be sought outside of the organisation and undertaken in personal time.

Strategies for personal development

Financial constraints and other challenges in health and social care provision may mean that CPD activities for support workers are not well promoted. In particular, this may apply to support workers where CPD is not mandatory for registration with a regulatory body. This places the onus squarely on the individual to determine strategies for personal development. Again, personal aspirations about future employment will inform thoughts about what those strategies might be. It may be that one-to-one conversations with a selected mentor may assist thinking about future roles, goals and CPD strategies. It is important that service constraints do not impact adversely on aspirations for personal advancement. There are other ways of planning to progress and achieve goals. After all, support workers are also entitled to a career. Many support workers apply to become professionally qualified once family commitments reduce giving more time for the necessary study. Support work at a steady pace in one locality may meet early needs but long-term goals should, wherever possible, be highlighted so that advantage can be taken of relevant CPD opportunities when they become available.

Keeping a personal portfolio

Employment opportunities can change quickly, especially in the light of economic downturns. Maintaining a CPD portfolio or profile is essential these days in order to be prepared for any change in the employment situation. Even if personal aspirations do not materialise and expectations have to change, any CPD activity undertaken, and any attempt in the pursuit of personal goals, will have enhanced personal capacity for alternative work. Additional qualifications may help and offer potential for other opportunities to be pursued. A belief in personal capability and the capacity to change direction in employment will also help. Keeping a portfolio of CPD activity and an up-to-date CV will ensure readiness for planned or unplanned changes in employment or unexpected employment opportunities.

Every support worker should be encouraged to keep a portfolio of professional development activities in the same way as their professionally qualified colleagues. Support workers unsure of how to create and use a portfolio to advantage should seek guidance. Colleagues will no doubt assist and there is further guidance in this book. Professional bodies can also be used as a resource, where appropriate. The choice of manual or electronic portfolio is up to the individual. There have been so many advances made in resources for portfolio management that many health professionals have moved to the electronic versions, but manual versions are simple and allow for recording much of the same information. However, an electronic version, for example PebblePad, is thought to be more flexible in its use, offering the ability to share observations and entries more easily with others, if that is desired. It is entirely the choice of the individual as to which version is selected as it is largely a resource for personal use.

An up-to-date portfolio can be drawn upon at any time to demonstrate CPD. Not only should it contain an up-to-date CV but also records of education and training undertaken that is particularly associated with the job. Records of new learning from different experiences are also useful and should include personal reflections on incidents that have led to learning and any further reading or research that has been undertaken following the learning experience. A future learning plan is also useful. Sometimes a portfolio is referred to as a personal learning journal as it records past learning experiences as a learning journey and reflects the impact of those experiences on the individual. The portfolio, or selected parts of it, can be referred to and can also be shared with others if desired. For example, parts of the portfolio may be relevant to support discussions at an appraisal or at any interview for advancement in the role or for entry to an educational programme.

Supervision and reflection on practice

Support workers must be supervised by a qualified member of a profession doing the same type of work. The supervisor, who is often the line manager, has a responsibility to nurture the development of the support worker as he or she makes a contribution to client care. The supervisor should assist the support worker in the process of reflection on interventions with, or for, service users, including those interventions that went well and those that did not go so well. Learning can derive from both. Initially, support workers may find it difficult to engage in this kind of retrospective review of their work to see how they can learn from experience. Supervisors should guide the process initially and suggest other activities that will assist learning. When the support worker is more confident, personal reflection on the way in which novel situations have been approached can be encouraged. Support workers should also expect to be included in other opportunities for reflection with professional staff to promote team learning. Some support workers are employed to work in a team and not specifically for a member of a named profession. For example, some support workers in health may assist both occupational therapists and physiotherapists in their work. Similarly, support workers in social care may make a contribution to the work of social workers and occupational therapists. Therefore, supervisors must give due consideration to the particular needs of the support worker in this role.

Assistant practitioners

The term support worker has initially been used as a generic term for unqualified staff performing duties in health and social care under the supervision of a regulated health professional. Some health professions have a designated role of Assistant Practitioner. Assistant practitioners are not regulated but have normally undertaken specific training in order to become competent to perform selected routine tasks under the supervision of the regulated professional. For example, the assistant practitioner in dietetics may be educated to Foundation Degree level and may deliver delegated dietetic care. Assistant practitioners in clinical imaging and radiotherapy will normally have studied to NVQ 3 or Foundation Degree level, or equivalent. After taking some accredited training specific to the role they may perform some limited examination or treatment procedures under supervision. Assistant technical officers work alongside biomedical scientists and can undertake specific duties. It might be envisaged that the number of assistant practitioners could well increase across the health care professions to maximise the use of expertise at different levels.

The Society and College of Radiographers has taken a lead in the United Kingdom to formalise career development opportunities within the profession from support workers to assistant practitioners, qualified practitioner, advanced practitioner and through to consultants and experts in the field. The College has produced an education and development strategy for the profession that acknowledges the various contributions to treatment and care management that each level of practitioner can make, some specifically under the supervision of registered radiographers. Scope and standards of work have been devised so that expectations are clear for the different clinical environments in which assistant practitioners might practise and relevant education requirements have been set. Accreditation rests with the College of Radiographers as no formal regulation by the Health and Care Professions Council (HCPC) is in place.

In order to remain competent in the role of assistant practitioner, ongoing learning and regular performance reviews should be expected. Clinical updating will be necessary as new procedures come into play and are adopted. Once the assistant practitioners appreciate the scope and potential of the work they do, they may opt to apply for relevant education and training to become formally qualified and eligible to apply for registration with the regulatory body. Keeping records of both formal and informal learning within a portfolio is essential to show how competence is being maintained and developed. An up-to-date portfolio will also support any application to a university and possibly to a fast-track qualifying course that takes account of previous qualifications and experience.

Working towards a professional qualification

Many support workers are happy in their role working with service users and administering tests, assessments or interventions according to a pre-defined protocol. However, some support workers may be attracted to the life of a qualified professional practising in health or social care. After a period of time in practice during which they gain relevant knowledge and experience of the role, support workers can take steps to secure a training place at university. A personalised CPD portfolio should support the application process as it helps demonstrate the capacity of the applicant to do the course. Most professional qualifying courses are full time but given the government's support for workplace learning, some qualifying programmes can be taken part time and some as work-based learning courses. Part-time courses enable students to continue in their regular employment on a part-time basis and to complete the qualifying course by studying for 2 or 3 days per week over an extended period of time. The combination of employment and study, with the demands of both simultaneously, will not meet everyone's needs even though the activities may be mutually supportive. Some people will prefer to study either full time or part time away from the distractions of work.

Finding a course that meets personal needs is key to success. Anyone thinking of applying for a professional qualifying programme should seek as much information as possible about potential courses and compare and contrast the different features. It should be possible to attend open days and to visit the course to gain some insights into the way in which the course is run and presented. Opportunities to speak to current students on the course should be explored. These activities will assist decision-making. The educational strategy used on the course will be important as they do vary, so it is wise to enquire about learning, teaching and assessment techniques that are used. Some courses may use a problem-based learning, enquiry-based learning or task-based learning strategy or pursue a more didactic approach. Each individual has preferred ways of learning, but on the course students will almost certainly be required to work and learn in a variety of ways both independently and in groups. Work-based learning courses are likely to follow 'situated learning' models with significant amounts of learning being derived from what is seen and practised in the workplace. These experiences must be reflected upon and discussed with colleagues and supervisors for relevant learning to occur. All professional courses expect students to master significant amounts of knowledge and theory to underpin practice and this can be quite challenging for those who have had a limited academic grounding and are more used to engaging with more practical tasks. However, perseverance will pay dividends.

Apart from the academic challenges, there are more practical issues to consider. Some applicants have family commitments, including the care of young children or elderly relatives. It is important to consider the timing of an application to pursue professional studies and how it fits in relation to other personal responsibilities. Personal health and stamina must be considered seriously as the course demands are significant. The geographical location of the course is also important as travelling is both costly and tiring. The relevant professional body will have information on its website about different courses leading to the professional qualification. The website of the selected university and its prospectus are other sources of information. All courses must be approved by the professional body, the regulatory body and the university so all will meet the required standards but the way in which this is done can vary considerably from university to university. The more information gathered about the course, the better informed will be the decision to apply for it. Becoming a qualified practitioner may be a long-term goal. As the decision to commit to the studies necessary to qualify is a significant one, it is worth talking to a course tutor about the expectations of the course so that any decision to apply for it is well informed.

Summary

This chapter has been dedicated specifically to the work and professional development of support workers. It is recognised amongst the professions in health and social care that the term support worker is generic and that those who hold such positions in employment may be known by a variety of different titles. Individuals who take employment as support workers do so for a variety of reasons. Whilst some remain in the role indefinitely, others may use it as a stepping stone for career development. Some may go on to attain specific qualifications to become assistant practitioners, others may seek a university place to study for a qualification in one of the health or social care professions. There are a number of different qualifying courses available and anyone seeking a place should evaluate the demands of the course and their own personal circumstances in order to maximise chances of success. Support workers are equally entitled to have opportunities for continuing professional development (CPD) in order to remain competent in their role. Some may be supported to gain recognised qualifications for advancement in their career. Maintaining an up-to-date portfolio is just as important for support workers as for professionally qualified personnel.

Chapter 14

Learning for leisure and pleasure

This chapter addresses:

1. ways in which leisure pursuits can be pleasurable for those taking breaks from employment or entering retirement;
2. opportunities for continuing lifelong learning in older age;
3. managing the transition to retirement.

Introduction

So far this book has promoted lifelong learning as an essential activity across the lifespan as a way of developing the skills necessary for personal and professional development and for competence in employment. The book has also tendered continuing professional development (CPD) as a necessary activity for professionals, students and support workers employed, or self-employed, in the delivery of health or social care to meet the need for best practice and public protection as required by regulatory bodies. However, at some time in life there may be breaks in employment and eventually working life will come to an end. The whole notion of lifelong learning is that throughout the lifespan learning continues and so keeps body and mind active and alert as new skills are developed. The need to acquire new skills throughout working life in order to meet new needs in changing circumstances has already been addressed. This chapter focuses on learning new knowledge and skills through leisure activities for health promotion and as a way of using time constructively in retirement.

Leisure

Leisure activities are inextricably linked to the health and well-being of both individuals and communities bringing a range of benefits to people of different ages across

---

Continuing Professional Development in Health and Social Care: Strategies for Lifelong Learning,
Second Edition. Auldeen Alsop.
© 2013 John Wiley & Sons, Ltd. Published 2013 by John Wiley & Sons, Ltd.

the lifespan. Leisure is seen as 'the time to engage freely in a chosen activity that brings value or positive outcomes to the individual' (Neumayer & Wilding, 2005, p. 319). Leisure activities are freely chosen for their own sake and not for employment, although they might include paid or unpaid work or other related activities. Learning to undertake new pursuits is often a feature of leisure activity as individuals take steps to acquire new skills in order to meet needs of self-expression and self-development (Christiansen & Townsend, 2004). Leisure activities can include a wide range of cultural practices, hobbies, outdoor pursuits as well as more sedentary activities such as craftwork, reading and listening to music. They often meet the need for self-expression and creativity. They may offer the time alone to escape from everyday responsibilities or they may offer a way of increasing social capital. Opportunities for developing new friends and companions through leisure pursuits can bring a sense of belonging to a group or community. Overall, leisure activities can enhance health and well-being often by countering some of the stresses and strains of everyday life. Leisure activities are exclusively for personal pleasure.

It is suggested that leisure activity is central to the human experience and that leisure can mean different things to different people (Thibodaux & Bundy, 1998). The meaning of the activity thus has particular significance for the individual. Leisure activities are distinguished from other activities as they are freely chosen and are totally under the control of the person engaging in them. They are also self-satisfying as engagement in the selected activity results in expression of individuality and a sense of accomplishment, thus promoting health. Many people are now seeing the benefits of spending more time on leisure pursuits to increase work-life balance. In this respect, some workers are now purposely reducing their hours of paid employment in order to increase their time available for more personally meaningful leisure pursuits, and so improve their quality of life. Reducing working hours could be the first step towards managing the retirement process.

Learning for pleasure

Learning is always the result of active occupation whether this takes place in formal or informal settings (Nelson & Jepson-Thomas, 2003). It can involve the acquisition of motor skills, cognitive skills or psychosocial skills and results in some new capacity to engage with the world. A lifetime of work can be devoted to learning new skills, updating knowledge and developing new ways of working as required of the employer. Learning for pleasure is purely a personal matter that brings more meaningful rewards to the individual. Space is hard to find in a busy working life to pursue more meaningful activities and bring balance to a lifestyle. However, as retirement approaches some more meaningful activities may begin to take centre stage. Learning for leisure opens up so many possibilities from sports groups, local interest groups to further education and to higher education through such organisations as the Open University. Also available for pursuing learning interests is the University of the Third Age known as the U3A (www.u3a.org.uk). This self-help organisation was established over 30 years ago for people no longer in employment. Those engaging with the U3A are those keen to pursue stimulating and creative leisure interests and opportunities that span the arts, history, philosophy, life sciences and many other creative and intellectual interests.

There are various organisations that help promote and guide lifelong learning by offering courses that stimulate and address the leisure interests of a retired population. Learning in older life helps develop new knowledge, maintain intellectual powers, create new interests and can enable the fulfilment of long-held ambitions. It offers personal stimulation, presents new challenges and prepares individuals for new adventures in later life.

Technology for learning

Health and social care professionals now entering retirement will almost certainly have developed a range of technological skills whilst in employment that will stand them in good stead as they retire. Computer technology, the Internet and an ever-increasing range of hand-held devices to aid communication have changed both working lives and personal lives quite significantly over the last few years and will continue to evolve at a considerable pace. Communication from home to local, national and international venues need never be a problem, so undertaking courses of interest or pursuing conversations and leisure activities with like-minded people across the world are now all possible. This adds a whole new dimension to leisure activity that can be home based yet interactive with anyone in the world. The term isolation has to be questioned as individuals operate alone in their own home yet communicate virtually with any number of people at significant distances across the planet. All these technological devices offer learning possibilities from the comfort of home. However, whilst many may use technology to communicate on a personal level, some may still enjoy learning in the presence of like-minded individuals who offer a different social dimension in reality.

Retirement

Retirement is one of the major transitions in life. The age of pensionable retirement is on the increase but individuals still have the choice to leave work earlier and pursue other activities. It may be possible to negotiate a graded transition from employment to retirement by reducing working hours over time. However, the key to a successful retirement is good planning. Loss of income will have a particular impact so financial matters such as pensions and mortgages need to be sorted out. Another significant loss will be a loss of structure to the working day, so giving consideration to constructive use of time after retirement will also aid the transition. Many large organisations offer pre-retirement courses and these tend to give sound advice about a range of important matters that are faced in the retirement years. Retirement can imply a loss, possibly of security, of income, or of a role in life, but if there is something new to look forward to, the feeling of loss could be minimised. In any transitional state there is a temporary period of adjustment that Bridges (1995) terms the neutral zone. It allows time for 'inner change' for things to sort themselves out, a time to take stock and make decisions about what the future should be. It can be a time for making creative decisions about ways of fulfilling other dreams. Possibilities are thus considered in a new light and with renewed vigour. New beginnings in retirement can then be tackled.

It has long been known that the number of older people in the population is growing at a significant pace and that retirement of those born in the 'baby boom' is now upon us adding to these growing numbers. Many health and social care professionals could fall within this group entering retirement over the next few years. These are skilled people, many of whom will take advantage of new free time to engage in chosen leisure pursuits. Others may seek meaningful activities that will lead them to make a particular contribution to their local community. Pilley (1993) saw the potential some years ago of taking steps to engage those recently retired, but still active people, in initiatives that would be of benefit to the community. Voluntary support groups for older people, younger people, for people with disabilities and for those convicted of offences offer potential opportunities. Other opportunities may be found through contact with religious organisations. Some roles will require individuals to undertake training, and once this is completed, the work can be allocated. Community work can be both challenging and satisfying, but it offers an avenue for using talent in a very different way to paid employment. Black and Living (2004) undertook research into volunteerism and its relationship to health and well-being. An analysis of some 109 questionnaires completed by volunteers indicated both altruistic and egoistic motivations for volunteering. Whilst there were some organisational issues that had to be tolerated, benefits included the social contact that volunteering offered and the opportunity to give something back to the community. Some negative experiences included frustration but others reported positive feelings indicating that volunteering contributed to emotional well-being.

Summary

This chapter has explored ways in which leisure pursuits can help maintain health and well-being and support a meaningful and productive life in retirement. Retirement is a life transition from work that brings opportunities for new ventures. Lifelong learning has been encouraged throughout this book but learning in retirement largely focuses on learning for pleasure. There are formal and informal ways in which learning can be continued in retirement. The use of technology can support the process. Retirement is a process that has to be managed and usually involves various stages of adjustment. Plans for a productive retirement that includes leisure pursuits, new learning goals or perhaps serving as a volunteer will assist the adjustment process and help maintain an active lifestyle in later life.

References

Black W & Living R (2004) Volunteerism as an occupation and its relationship to health and wellbeing. *British Journal of Occupational Therapy*, **67** (12), 526–532.
Bridges W (1995) *Managing Transitions*. Nicholas Brealey Publishing, London.

Christiansen CH & Townsend EA (2004) *Introduction to Occupation, the Art and Science of Living*. Prentice Hall, Upper Saddle River, NJ.

Nelson D & Jepson-Thomas J (2003) Occupational form, occupational performance, and a conceptual framework for therapeutic occupation. In: *Perspectives in Human Occupation* (eds P Kramer, J Hinojosa & CB Royeen), pp. 87–155. Lippincott Williams and Wilkins, Baltimore, MD.

Neumayer B & Wilding C (2005) Leisure as commodity. In: *Occupation & Practice in Context* (eds G Whiteford & V Wright-St Clair), pp. 317–331. Elsevier Churchill Livingstone, Sydney.

Pilley C (1993) Adult education, community development and older people. In: *Adult Learners, Education and Training* (eds R Edwards, S Sieminski & D Zeldin), pp. 265–276. Routledge in association with the Open University, London.

Thibodaux LR & Bundy AC (1998) Leisure. In: *Sociology & Occupational Therapy: An Integrated Approach* (eds D Jones, SEE Blair, T Hartery & RK Jones), pp. 157–170. Churchill Livingstone, Edinburgh.

Index

academic careers 125–35
  career development 125–35
  continuing careers in academia 127–9
  early academic careers 126–7
  keeping in touch with practice
    129–30
  research 93–4, 131, 132–4
  service learning and community
    engagement 130–1, 133
  UK Professional Standards
    Framework 128–9
accreditation of prior learning (APL)
  72, 98–9
accredited learning in the workplace
  73–5, 81
achievement coaching 41
action learning 141–2, 145
active listening/questioning 41–2, 62
advanced practice 118–19, 123
analytical skills 4
assistant practitioners 150–1
audits
  leadership 138
  learning to learn 54
  professional portfolios 26–7
  regulatory factors 18–21
  writing skills 102, 105
authorship 65–6
autonomous learners 48–9, 56
autonomous practitioners 51–2, 56

bachelor's degrees 84, 87–8, 94–5
Bologna Process 87

book reviews 110–11
breaks from practice 31–2, 96, 122

career development 114–24
  academic careers 125–35
  advanced practice 118–19, 123
  advancing in a career 117–19
  career choices 119–20
  continuing careers in academia
    127–9
  definitions and characteristics 115–16
  early academic careers 126–7
  keeping in touch with practice
    129–30
  mentorship 117, 121–2
  opportunities and approaches 116–17
  practical steps 122–3
  professional isolation 120–2
  research 93–4, 117, 131, 132–4
  service learning and community
    engagement 130–1, 133
  UK Professional Standards
    Framework 128–9
career enhancement 17–18
career planning
  learning careers 38, 44–5
  practical steps 122–3
  professional portfolios 32–3
case studies 103
Chartered Institute of Personnel
  Development (CIPD) 9
co-learners 121–2
coaching 40–2

Continuing Professional Development in Health and Social Care: Strategies for Lifelong Learning,
Second Edition. Auldeen Alsop.
© 2013 John Wiley & Sons, Ltd. Published 2013 by John Wiley & Sons, Ltd.

Codes of Ethics and Professional
    Conduct 14
collaborative learning 58–67
    career development 120–1
    critical kinship 62–3, 64
    learning events 60–1
    mechanisms for supported learning
        62–5
    participatory action research 61
    projects in partnership 59–62
    publication 65–6
    social spaces 64–5
    storytelling 61–2, 66
    workplace learning 79, 80
Commonwealth Scholarship
    Commission 80–1
communication skills
    collaborative learning 60
    learning careers 37
    lifelong learning 3–4
    pleasure 155
    workplace learning 70
    see also writing skills
communities
    collaborative learning 58–9
    engagement with 130–1, 133
    of learning 79
    leisure activities 153–4
    retirement 156
competence to practice
    higher education 84
    learning careers 36–7
    learning to learn 47, 50–1, 56
    lifelong learning 7–9
    regulatory factors 15, 18–19
conferences 43, 60–1
conflicts of interest 74–5
consultancy 30, 119
Council for Graduate Education 74
creative writing 26, 112
creativity
    career development 117–18
    leadership 143
    lifelong learning 4
    workplace learning 76–7
critical appraisal and evaluation 86

critical companionship 64, 122
critical incidents 106
critical kinship 62–3, 64
critical reflection 52, 85, 96
critical writing 107, 110–11, 112
curriculum vitae (CV) 27, 29–32,
    122–3, 149

decision-making skills
    learning careers 35
    learning to learn 52
    support workers 151
    writing skills 106
delegation 141
development plans 38–9, 44–5
diplomas 84, 85, 94–5
distance learning 87, 94–5
doctorates 74, 81, 84, 87–9, 91–3, 119

e-learning
    higher education 87
    leadership 139
    workplace learning 71–2
e-portfolios 24, 25, 30, 149
early learning 47–8, 56
educational programmes 80, 87, 132
emotional support 42, 43
employability
    career development 115
    lifelong learning 3–4
    workplace learning 80
enterprise 4, 55
envisioning a career 36
Erasmus programme 132
ethics
    leadership 142
    lifelong learning 6–7
    regulatory factors 14
    support workers 146
European Network of Occupational
    Therapy in Higher Education
    (ENOTHE) 132
European Platform for Worldwide
    Social Work (EUSW) 132
European Qualifications Framework for
    Lifelong Learning 87–8

evidence 23, 26–7, 39
experiential learning
  higher education 96–7, 98–9
  leadership 142
  learning to learn 52, 53, 56
  workplace learning 69–70, 76
expertise
  career development 119–20
  higher education 86–7
  leadership 144
  learning to learn 49–50, 55

formal learning
  learning to learn 48
  lifelong learning 2
  pre-registration learning 15–16
  workplace learning 70–2
Foundation Degrees 150
funding
  career development 131–2
  lifelong learning 10
  regulatory factors 18
  workplace learning 77

graduate portfolios 27–8
grants 132
group membership 3, 28
Grundtvig scheme 132

Health and Care Professions Council
    (HCPC)
  career development 120, 125, 128–9
  higher education 96
  leadership 144
  lifelong learning 8, 9–10
  professional portfolios 23, 26–7,
    31–3
  regulatory factors 8, 13–15, 18–21
  support workers 151
  workplace learning 72–3
helicopter vision 3
higher education 84–100
  academic careers 93–4, 125–35
  accreditation of prior learning 98–9
  career development 119, 125–35
  expectations and ownership 97

experiential learning 96–7, 98–9
independent study 96–7
knowledge, skills and competence 89
learning preferences 94–7
mode of learning 94–5
motivations and outcomes 85–7
pleasure 154
professional doctorates 92–3
research degrees 88, 90–1
returning to learning 95–6
taught higher degrees 92
transfer to PhD 91
typical qualifications 87–93
workplace learning 73, 81
writing skills 109–10, 111
Higher Education Academy (HEA)
    128–9
Higher National Diploma (HND) 87,
    88

incidental learning 2
independent study 96–7
individual performance reviews (IPR)
    43–5, 55, 71
informal learning
  learning to learn 54
  lifelong learning 2
  workplace learning 70–1, 72
  see also experiential learning
information leaflets 110
information literacy 3
innovation 78, 139, 143
interpersonal skills 3
  see also communication skills
interviews 29–30

Johns' model for structured reflection
    53–4
journaling 26, 104–5, 112, 140–1

Knowledge and Skills Framework 40

lead authors 65
leadership 136–45
  action learning 141–2, 145
  attributes of leaders 138–9

leadership (*Continued*)
  career development 119, 129
  definitions and characteristics 136–7
  development of leadership skills
    139–40
  expertise 144
  innovation 139, 143
  management development 137–8
  organisational change 142–3
  support for aspiring leaders 141
  transition to leader 140–1
learning careers 34–46
  coaching and mentorship 40–2
  developing competence 36–7
  envisioning a career 36
  individual performance reviews 43–5
  networks 42–3
  performance reviews/appraisals 36,
    37–8, 43–5
  preceptorship 38, 39–40
  process of CPD 37–43
  professional journeys 34–6
  reflective skills 39, 41–3
learning events 60–1
learning organisations 58–9, 60, 127
learning outcomes 102–3
learning partnerships 58, 59–62
learning skills 36
learning strategies 146–52
learning to learn 47–57
  autonomous learners 48–9, 56
  autonomous practitioners 51–2, 56
  competence to practice 47, 50–1, 56
  early learning 47–8, 56
  experiential learning 52, 53, 56
  identifying learning needs 49–50
  learning as an investment 55
  reflection 52–6
  stages of professional development
    49–50
  student learners 48–9
lectureships 125–8
leisure activities 153–4, 156
lifelong learning 1–11
  competence to practice 7–9
  context 1–2

continuing professional development
  1–2, 9–10
  definitions and characteristics 2–3
  employability 3–4
  ethics and quality of care delivery 6–7
  higher education 87–8
  leadership 144
  learning careers 36
  learning to learn 48
  pleasure 155
  portfolio careers 5–6
  professional careers 4–6, 7–9
  regulatory factors 8, 16, 17
  workplace learning 80
literature reviews 111
long-term objectives 37–8

management careers 85, 118
  see also leadership
manual portfolios 24–5, 30, 149
Master of Business Administration
  (MBA) 85, 119, 137
Master of Philosophy (MPhil) 88, 90–1
Master's degrees 73, 81, 84, 85, 87–92,
  119
mentorship
  career development 117, 121–2
  collaborative learning 64
  leadership 137, 141
  learning careers 40–2
  support workers 148
  workplace learning 74
multidisciplinary teams 42–3, 71, 79

National Health Service (NHS) 40, 80,
  140
national register 13–14
National Vocational Qualifications
  (NVQ) 71, 147
networks
  career development 121–2
  learning careers 42–3
  learning to learn 51
neutral zone 155–6
new graduate portfolios 27–8
novice-to-expert continuum 49–50

occupational therapy 40, 150
Occupational Therapy International
    Outreach Network (OTION) 121
organisational change 142–3
organisational culture 79
organisational learning 58–9, 60, 127
organisational objectives 41

part-time employment 4–5
participatory action research 61
partnerships 58, 59–62
PebblePad 24, 25, 102, 149
peer support networks 43, 121–2
performance reviews/appraisals 43–5
    collaborative learning 62, 64
    learning to learn 55
    process of CPD 36, 37–8
    support workers 147–8
    workplace learning 71
personal agency 3
personal appraisals *see* individual
    performance reviews
personal development
    career development 116–17
    collaborative learning 59
    higher education 86
    leadership 141
    learning careers 36–7
    learning to learn 47–8, 55–6
    leisure activities 153–4, 156
    lifelong learning 3, 6
    pleasure 154–5
    retirement 155–6
    support workers 148–50
    workplace learning 77–9
    writing skills 102–3
personal objectives 41
physiotherapy 150
placements 68
pleasure 154–5
portfolio careers 5–6
postgraduate certificates 88, 89–90, 127
post-qualification career paths 35
post-registration learning 69
practitioner portfolios 28–9
preceptorship 38, 39–40, 69

pre-registration learning 15–16, 68
presentation history 28
private practice 30
problem-solving skills 3–4, 141–2, 143
professional bodies
    career development 129
    higher education 86–7
    professional portfolios 28, 29
    support workers 146, 149
professional careers 4–6, 7–9
professional doctorates 74, 81, 84,
    92–3, 119
professional isolation 120–2
professional journeys 34–6
professional portfolios 22–33
    breaks from and returning to practice
        31–2
    career development 125
    compilation and development of 30–1
    definitions and characteristics 22–3
    e-portfolios 24, 25, 30
    evidence and profiles 23, 26–7
    higher education 84
    interviews and promotions 28, 29–30
    journaling and creative writing 26
    leadership 140
    manual portfolios 24–5, 30
    new graduate portfolios 27–8
    practitioner portfolios 28–9
    professional development and career
        planning 32–3
    prospective and retrospective
        approaches 31
    regulatory factors 23, 26–7, 31–3
    scrapbooking 25–6
    student portfolios 27
    support workers 149, 151
    variations of portfolio 23–7
    workplace learning 75–6
    writing skills 102, 107
professional qualifications 7–9
profiles 23, 26–7
project proposals 103–4
promotions 28, 29–30, 38
proposals 103–4
prospective approaches 31

protean careers 4, 117
publication
    collaborative learning 65–6
    professional portfolios 28
    writing skills 109, 111–13

quality of care delivery 6–7

radiography 150–1
reasoning skills 50–1
reflection
    collaborative learning 63, 66
    higher education 85, 96
    learning careers 39, 41–3
    learning to learn 52–6
    support workers 150
    workplace learning 69–70, 75–6
    writing skills 101, 104–7, 112
regulatory factors 12–21
    career development 114, 120, 125,
        127–9
    career enhancement 17–18
    competence to practice 15, 18–19
    expectations of practitioners 14–15
    experience of audit 20–1
    leadership 138, 144
    learning careers 39, 45
    learning to learn 54
    lifelong learning 8, 16, 17
    meeting regulatory requirements
        18–19
    national register 13–14
    pre-registration education 15–16
    professional portfolios 23, 26–7,
        31–3
    specific CPD requirements 14
    submissions for CPD audit 19–21
    support workers 148, 150–1
    United Kingdom context 13–15,
        18–21
    workplace learning 72–3, 76, 79–80
    writing skills 102, 105
research
    career development 93–4, 117, 131,
        132–4
    conflicts of interest 74–5

higher education 86, 90–4
    professional portfolios 20, 28
    workplace learning 74–5
    writing skills 109–10, 111
retirement 154, 155–6
retrospective approaches 31
returning to learning 95–6
returning to practice 31–2
reviews 107, 109–11

sabbaticals 131–2
scrapbooking 25–6
secondments 142
security
    career development 114–16
    learning to learn 55
    lifelong learning 5
    workplace learning 77
self-employment 6, 119–20, 125
self-evaluation 49, 54–5
self-management skills 4
service learning 130–1
shadowing experts 76
shared authorship 65–6
short-term objectives 38
situated learning 152
Skill Acquisition Model 49–50
social learning 79
social media 51
social spaces 64–5
social workers 73, 150
Society and College of Radiographers
    150–1
specialisation
    career development 119–20, 127–8
    higher education 85
    learning careers 38, 43
    learning to learn 49–50
    support workers 148
specialist interest groups 59
sponsorship 18, 131–2
storytelling 61–2, 66
structured reflection 53–4
student learners 48–9
student portfolios 27
study days 60

supervision
  collaborative learning 62, 64
  learning careers 36
  support workers 150
  writing skills 110
support workers
  assistant practitioners 150–1
  learning strategies 146–52
  performance reviews/appraisals
    147–8
  personal expectations and aspirations
    147–8
  professional portfolios 149, 151
  professional qualification 151–2
  strategies for personal development
    148–50
  supervision and reflection on practice
    150
supported learning 62–5, 121–2

teaching qualifications 85, 127
team awaydays 60
teamwork
  career development 120–1
  leadership 140
  learning careers 42–3
  lifelong learning 3–4
  workplace learning 71, 79
technology
  career development 114
  collaborative learning 60
  learning careers 43
  learning to learn 51, 56
  lifelong learning 4
  pleasure 155
teleconferencing 43
Tuning programme 80

UK Professional Standards Framework
  (UKPSF) 128–9
unpaid work experience 27, 30

voluntary work
  professional portfolios 27, 30
  retirement 156
  workplace learning 77

Whole Systems Thinking/Development
  61
work experience 27, 30
work–life balance 4–5, 154
workplace learning 68–83
  accredited learning in the workplace
    73–5, 81
  communities of learning 79
  conflicts of interest 74–5
  experiential learning 69–70, 76
  formal and informal learning
    70–2
  higher education 87
  international perspectives 79–81
  learning types 69
  making the most of 75–7
  organisational culture 79
  social workers 73
  transforming ourselves 77–9
  transforming practice 78–9
workshops 61
writing skills 101–13
  case studies 103
  creative writing 26, 112
  critical incidents 106
  critical writing 107, 110–11,
    112
  journaling 104–5, 112
  learning events 105–6
  personal challenge 107–8
  personal development plans
    102–3
  project proposals 103–4
  public audiences 109–12
  reflection 101, 104–7, 112
  style and identity 108–9